Problems and Solutions

SURGERY

**Revision questions
in undergraduate surgery**

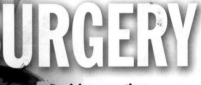

Editors

Andrew Goldberg
The Nuffield Orthopaedic Centre
Oxford, UK

Gerard Stansby
Newcastle University & Freeman Hospital
Newcastle Hospitals NHS Trust, UK

Problems and Solutions

SURGERY

Revision questions
in undergraduate surgery

Imperial College Press

ICP

Published by

Imperial College Press
57 Shelton Street
Covent Garden
London WC2H 9HE

Distributed by

World Scientific Publishing Co. Pte. Ltd.
5 Toh Tuck Link, Singapore 596224
USA office: 27 Warren Street, Suite 401-402, Hackensack, NJ 07601
UK office: 57 Shelton Street, Covent Garden, London WC2H 9HE

British Library Cataloguing-in-Publication Data
A catalogue record for this book is available from the British Library.

SURGERY: PROBLEMS AND SOLUTIONS
Revision Questions in Undergraduate Surgery

ISBN-13 978-1-84816-187-0 (pbk)
ISBN-10 1-84816-187-5 (pbk)

Typeset by Stallion Press
Email: enquiries@stallionpress.com

Printed in Singapore by Mainland Press Pte Ltd

About the Authors

Gerard Stansby, MB, MCHir, FRCS

Professor Gerard Stansby qualified from Cambridge University and Addenbrooke's Hospital in 1982. He carried out many junior training posts in Cambridge and the East Anglian area before moving to the Royal Free Hospital as Registrar and subsequently Lecturer in Surgery. In 1993, he went to St. Mary's Hospital in London as a Senior Clinical Vascular Fellow and, in 1994, became Senior Lecturer in General and Vascular Surgery at St. Mary's Hospital and Imperial College, London. In January 2000, he obtained his current position of Professor of Vascular Surgery at the Freeman Hospital, University of Newcastle.

Professor Stansby is the author of more than 150 scientific articles and several books and book chapters. His special interests include platelet–blood vessel wall and vascular risk factors. He is co-chair of the TARGET-PAD group which aims to improve the profile and understanding of PAD in the UK, a Council member of the Vascular Society of Great Britain and Ireland, a Council member of the Venous Forum and an editor for the Cochrane Peripheral Vascular Diseases group and several medical journals. He has been an examiner for final medical students at several medical schools in the UK and overseas and chairs the Newcastle Surgical Undergraduate Teaching Committee.

Andrew Goldberg, MBBS, MD, FRCS (Tr&Orth)

Mr. Goldberg qualified from the Imperial College School of Medicine in 1994. His specialist training was based on the Royal National Orthopaedic Hospital, Stanmore and Royal Free Hospital Orthopaedic training programme in the North East Thames Region. He is a fellow of the Royal College of Surgeons of England and Ireland and a member of the British Orthopaedic Association. He obtained his CCT in Trauma and Orthopaedics in 2007 and now specialises in lower limb surgery. Andy founded the Medical Futures Innovation Awards in 2001, which is one of the UK's highest healthcare accolades and assists medical professionals progress their innovative ideas closer to implementation and patient benefit. Andy authored a paper for the Parliamentary under Secretary of State for Health entitled, "Encouraging, Supporting and Rewarding Innovation in the NHS" in 2004 and was also a member of the DTi led Health Industries Taskforce (HITF). In 2007, Andy was invited to sit on the UK Department of Health's Innovation Council. Andy coined the term "ideapreneurs" and speaks regularly at national and international meetings on the subject of healthcare innovation. Andy has an MD thesis on cartilage repair, based on pioneering work in human mesenchymal stem cells. He also enjoys teaching medical students and finding ways to help convey complex issues in easy to understand and memorable ways.

Acknowledgements

To our parents and wives who are always there for us and always a forethought. To our amazing children who give us reason to teach, share knowledge and enjoy what we do.
To all the contributing authors who brought their invaluable depth of expertise. To all of the medical students, for their suggestions before and after the book was written.

Preface

It is important to explain at the outset that we do not regard this as a typical "test yourself" book. There are no pass marks and it is not designed as a set of mock-exam questions with model answers. We regard it as a way of learning or revising a topic, by challenging yourself. The best approach is to attempt a question and then use the answers provided to test or supplement your knowledge. We believe that putting the answers immediately after the questions will suit many students far better than the approach of most other revision aids, where the answers are hidden at the back. We would suggest you answer one question at a time (with the answers covered) and then consider the given answer, before moving to the next question. But of course it is your book — so you may do as you please! Obviously, a revision aid cannot be exhaustive and so depending on your background level of knowledge you may also wish to look up some points in a standard text book before moving on. We have used the "single best answer" format in the MCQ's and EMQ's as this appears to be in use in the majority of medical schools at the present time. We hope that this format will result in an understanding of context as well as the retention of facts.

Deliberately we have not linked the current book with our previous text book "Surgical Talk", as we felt students would wish to have completely fresh stand-alone text. Of course there will be a large amount of overlap, but we make no apologies for the fact that a few topics or answers may be found in one book but not the other. However, as with "Surgical Talk", this book aims for a level of knowledge and the approach that would be expected of the better students arriving at finals. Some of the questions are deliberately quite difficult — but we hope all are fair! Like "Surgical Talk" we have also included ENT, orthopaedics and urology as well as general surgery so that you do not have to buy endless revision aids to ensure you have surgery covered.

Finally we would like to thank our colleagues and friends who have contributed the questions and answers. They are all very busy people and so we are very grateful for their help.

Good luck with your revision and the exam. We hope this book will help you prepare for surgical finals with enthusiasm and confidence.

Gerard Stansby
Andrew Goldberg

Contributors

Muhammad Ishtiaq Ahmed, MRCS
*Clinical Research Fellow, School of Surgical and Reproductive Sciences,
Newcastle University, UK*

Douglas Aitken, FRCS (Gen Surg)
*Specialist Registrar, Colorectal Surgery, Royal Victoria Infirmary,
Newcastle-upon-Tyne, UK*

Ben Bannerjee, MD, FRCS
*Consultant Surgeon and Honorary Senior Lecturer, Sunderland Royal Hospitals,
Sunderland, UK*

Sheila Carey, FRCA
Specialist Registrar in Anaesthetics, Northern Deanery, UK

Richard M. Charnley, DM, FRCS
*Consultant Hepato-Pancreato-Biliary Surgeon, Freeman Hospital,
Newcastle-upon-Tyne, UK*

Joseph Cosgrove, FRCA
Consultant Anaesthetist, Freeman Hospital, Newcastle-upon-Tyne, UK

Praveen Dadireddy, MRCS
Trainee, ENT, Pilgrim Hospital, Boston, Lincolnshire, UK

S. Michael Griffin, MD, FRCS, FRCS Ed, FCS (HK)
*Professor of Gastrointestinal Surgery, Northern Oesophagogastric Unit,
Royal Victoria Infirmary, Newcastle-upon-Tyne, UK*

Monica Hansrani, MD, FRCS
Specialist Registrar, Vascular Surgery, Northern Deanery, UK

Alan F. Horgan, MD, FRCS
Consultant Colorectal Surgeon, Freeman Hospital, Newcastle-upon-Tyne, UK

Smout Jonathan, MD FRCS
Specialist Registrar, Vascular Surgery, Newcastle-upon-Tyne, UK

Nigel Jones, MS, FRCS
Consultant Surgeon, Freeman Hospital, Newcastle-upon-Tyne, UK

Tom Lennard, MD, FRCS
Professor of Breast and Endocrine Surgery and Head of School,
School of Surgical and Reproductive Sciences,
Newcastle University, UK

Rajiv Lochan, MS, FRCSEd
Specialist Registrar, Hepatobiliary Surgery, Freeman Hospital,
Newcastle-upon-Tyne, UK

Roy McGregor, BSc(Hons), FRCS(Urol)
Fellow in Urology, The Royal North Shore Hospital, Sydney, Australia

Ashraf Morgan, MS, FRCS
Staff Grade Surgeon, Pilgrim Hospital, Boston, Lincolnshire, UK

Ian Nesbitt, FRCA, Dip. ICM
Consultant Anaesthetist, Freeman Hospital, Newcastle-upon-Tyne, UK

Michael Oko, FRCS
Consultant ENT Surgeon, Pilgrim Hospital, Boston, Lincolnshire, UK

Klaus Overbeck, FRCS
Consultant Vascular Surgeon, Sunderland Royal Hospitals, Sunderland, UK

Dorota Overbeck-Zubrzycka, MD
Specialist Surgical Trainee, Northern Deanery, UK

Rehan Saif, MRCS
Clinical Research Fellow, School of Surgical and Reproductive Sciences,
Newcastle University, UK

Christopher Streets, BSc, MD, FRCS (Gen Surg)
Consultant, Department of Surgery, Bristol Royal Infirmary, UK

Contents

Chapter 1   Trauma, Shock, Head Injuries and Burns

Sheila Carey and Jonathan Smout

Multiple Choice Questions

[*Each single best answer (SBA) question comprises a stem and a number of answers. You are asked to decide which single item represents the best answer to the question.*]

1. **The primary survey in trauma**

    a) Aims to identify all injuries
    b) Should be completed before instituting any treatment
    c) Staff must take relevant precautions to protect themselves
    d) Should be performed only once
    e) Includes AP X-rays of the c-spine, chest and pelvis

[Best Answer = c]

Explanation

The primary survey is intended to identify immediately life-threatening injuries in a systematic manner. It is broken down into steps which you will know as ABCDE (Airway, Breathing, Circulation, Disability, and Exposure). Appropriate diagnostic and resuscitative methods are employed simultaneously. Protection of the medical staff against communicable diseases is of paramount importance and a face mask, eye protection, water impervious apron and gloves should be considered minimum precautions. The patient should be constantly re-assessed to evaluate response to resuscitation. By repeating the primary survey regularly any deterioration in the patient's condition is noted and acted upon quickly. The secondary survey is a head-to-toe evaluation of the patient which begins only when the primary survey is complete, resuscitation well established with a return towards normalisation of the patients vital signs. A lateral c-spine, AP chest and AP pelvis are the initial trauma X-ray series carried out during the primary survey.

2. Haemorrhage

a) Palpable carotid pulsation indicates normo-volaemia
b) Thirty per cent of circulating blood volume may be lost without changes in blood pressure
c) Leads to a decreased conscious level at an early stage
d) Normal capillary refill is > 2 seconds
e) Blood pressure is a good measure of tissue perfusion

[Best Answer = b]

Explanation

The human body's ability to compensate for fluid shifts is remarkable. Major organ perfusion is maintained by vasoconstriction of non-vital tissues such as the skin and splanchnic circulation, combined with an increase in cardiac rate and contractility. By the time hypo-volaemia affects the cerebral circulation, and lowers the conscious level it will have reached a critical level. Haemorrhagic shock is "inadequate tissue perfusion and tissue oxygenation" as a result of haemorrhage. Perfusion is not synonymous with blood pressure and can be compromised before blood pressure falls. There are four stages of shock based on the percentage of blood loss as per the following table.

During stage I and II shock, the conscious level may be heightened.

Stage	Stage I	Stage II	Stage III	Stage IV
Blood loss (%)	<15%	15%–30%	30%–40%	>40%
Blood loss (ml)	<750	750–1500	1500–2000	>2000
Consciousness	Slightly anxious	Agitated	Confused	Depressed
Pulse rate	<100	>100	>120	>140
Blood pressure	Normal	Normal	Decreased	Decreased
Pulse pressure	Normal	Decreased	Decreased	Decreased
Respiratory rate	14–20	20–30	30–40	>35
Urine output (ml/h)	>30	20–30	5–15	Negligible
Replacement	Crystalloid	Colloid	Colloid + Blood	Colloid + Blood

3. **Cervical spine assessment**

   a) Adequate cervical spine (c-spine) immobilisation is obtained with either a hard collar or a spinal board head box
   b) A normal lateral c-spine X-ray can exclude c-spine injury
   c) The pre-vertebral tissue in the upper c-spine should be >5 mm on a lateral c-spine film
   d) Swimmers view always shows the C7-T1 junction adequately
   e) Intervertebral discs should be approximately of equal height

[Best Answer = e]

Explanation

C-spine assessment is often difficult in the acute situation where conscious level is altered and multiple injuries are present. Mechanical immobilisation of the c-spine requires a hard collar plus sand bags and tape or a head box. Clearing the c-spine in the emergency room requires a satisfactory clinical examination plus adequate c-spine radiology (C1-T1) and even then in cases of suspicion further imaging might be necessary. There should be a high index of suspicion of injury in multi-system trauma particularly if there is blunt injury above the clavicles. The pre-vertebral soft tissue in the upper c-spine should measure <5 mm, swelling in this area can signify underlying bony or ligamentous injury. Downward traction of the arms for lateral X-ray or a swimmers view aids visualising the C7-T1 junction but in some cases an adequate view cannot be obtained with plain X-rays and a CT scan is indicated.

4. **Fluid replacement and venous access in trauma**

   a) Central venous cannulation is essential for initial fluid replacement in trauma
   b) Venous cannulae flow rates increase in a linear fashion with the radius
   c) Resuscitation fluids should be warmed to 60°C
   d) Hartmann's solution (Ringers lactate) should be given carefully due to its potassium content
   e) The internal jugular vein usually lies lateral to the carotid artery in the neck

[Best Answer = e]

Explanation

> The flow rate of any tube is proportional to the fourth power of the radius. Hence, a central venous catheter (a long thin tube), whilst is useful to measure fluid status, is not ideal to replace fluid quickly. In contrast, a thick bore peripheral IV cannula (short and thick) is quicker to insert and has much better flow characteristics. Warmed fluids are important to prevent hypothermia and the temperature should ideally be 37°C–40°C. Hartmann's solution has a physiological potassium concentration and therefore will not induce acute hyperkalaemia with rapid infusion.

5. With regard to airway assessment in trauma

a) If a patient is talking, the assessor can move on to C for circulation.
b) Airway compromise should be suspected if noisy breathing is present
c) All trauma patients require intubation
d) C-spine control is only required if the patient has neck pain
e) Immobilisation devices should not be removed from the c-spine to facilitate intubation

[Best Answer = b]

Explanation

> An unobstructed airway is paramount to facilitate delivery of oxygen. Patency must be ascertained before anything else and the ABC rule should always be followed. Airway obstruction can be partial or complete and may be associated with snoring, gurgling or stridor. Simple measures such as chin lift, jaw thrust and use of airway adjuncts such as a Guedel or nasopharyngeal airways may be sufficient to relieve obstruction, whilst c-spine stabilisation is maintained at the same time. A c-spine injury should be suspected in anyone with altered consciousness, injuries above the clavicles or where the history is suggestive of potential injury. Stabilisation equipment should be left in place until injury is excluded but may be removed temporarily to facilitate intubation providing manual in-line immobilisation of the head and neck is maintained.

6. Regarding chest drain insertion

a) Should be inserted in the mid-axillary line in the fifth intercostal space
b) When creating a track for the drain, keep close to the undersurface of the rib
c) It is the initial treatment for a tension pneumothorax
d) Asepsis can be overlooked in the trauma situation
e) A 12-French gauge (12G or 12F) drain is satisfactory for a tension pneumothorax

[Best Answer = a]

Explanation

The fifth intercostal space in the mid-axillary line is a safe site for chest drain insertion bilaterally. The neurovascular bundle of each rib lies in a groove on its undersurface; hence, the drain track should run on the upper surface of the rib. The initial management of a tension pneumothorax is by needle decompression. Preparation and insertion of a chest drain is not an instantaneous process and will often take longer than expected particularly in inexperienced hands. Standard aseptic techniques should still be used despite the hurried situation. A pneumothorax will be adequately drained with a 24G drain, however in the case where a haemothorax is present a larger size of drain (38G) is often more effective.

7. Regarding the physiology of head injuries

a) The skull vault allows for expansion as intracranial bleeding occurs
b) The normal intracranial pressure is usually close to the mean arterial pressure
c) It is possible to accommodate a mass of up to 100 ml without a significant raise in ICP
d) Increasing arterial pCO_2 causes cerebral vasoconstriction
e) Cerebral perfusion pressure = mean arterial pressure + the intracranial pressure

[Best Answer = c]

Explanation

The skull vault is a rigid cavity of a fixed volume. It contains brain, blood and cerebrospinal fluid (CSF) and increasing the volume of any one component will thus lead to a reduction in another or intracranial pressure will increase (Monroe-Kellie Doctrine). The cerebral perfusion pressure equals the mean arterial pressure minus the intracranial pressure; hence increasing the MAP or decreasing the intracranial pressure improves cerebral perfusion. Increasing levels of arterial CO_2 results in vasodilatation and should be avoided in the head injured patient.

8. Extradural haemorrhage

a) Is usually associated with a skull fracture
b) Often involves disruption of the middle cerebral artery
c) Loss of consciousness always occurs at the time of injury
d) Falling intracranial pressure leads to herniation of the uncus through the tentorium
e) Hemiparesis and third cranial nerve injury are both on the contralateral side

[Best Answer = a]

Explanation

Extradural haemorrhage occurs secondary to bleeding from the arteries supplying the skull. On CT there is typically a high density lens-shaped lesion on the inner surface of the skull. The middle meningeal artery is usually disrupted from a fracture in the temporal region of the skull. There is typically a brief loss of consciousness followed by a lucid interval. During this lucid interval the haematoma is expanding into the extradural space and compressing the brain inwards, stripping the dura off the skull as it expands (hence the convex appearance of the clot on the CT). The intracranial pressure (ICP) does not rise initially as the mass is accommodated; however, once the clot reaches a critical volume the ICP increases rapidly, causing a secondary lapse in the consciousness level. As the ICP rises further the uncus (the medial aspect of the temporal lobe) herniates through the tentorium (the layer that divides the cerebral hemispheres from the brain stem and cerebellum). The third nerve passes through this opening and can be compressed at this point. The patient initially develops a constriction of the pupil on the affected side, which then begins to dilate up (Hutchinson's pupil). The fixed dilated pupil on the affected side is usually accompanied by a hemiparesis on the opposite side (remember the corticospinal fibres cross over). As the pressure continues to increase, the opposite pupil dilates up and eventually the brain stem "cones" through the foramen magnum.

9. Management of a burns patient

a) Carbon monoxide (CO) levels are rarely measured
b) CO-haemoglobin levels of >5% on arrival at hospital suggest serious poisoning
c) Circulatory optimisation for fluid losses takes priority over airway management
d) Increasing the inspired O_2 concentration reduces CO-haemoglobin half-life
e) Cherry red skin colouration is common in CO poisoning

[Best Answer = d]

Explanation

CO poisoning should be considered in all patients suspected of inhalation injury and those who have suffered burns in an enclosed area and such patients require CO measurement. Significant airway injury is suggested by facial burns, respiratory distress, inflammation/oedema of the mouth or oropharynx, hoarse voice, singed nasal hairs and carbonaceous sputum. An initial patent airway in this situation can be compromised as swelling develops, so early involvement of an anaesthetist is mandatory. CO-haemoglobin levels of >15% on arrival at hospital suggest serious poisoning. CO has a higher affinity for haemoglobin but its half-life can be reduced by giving high flow O_2. It should be remembered that the arterial oxygen concentration does not predict CO poisoning. Cherry red skin colouration is rarely seen.

10. Burns

a) One per cent of a patients body surface (BSA) area equates to the size of your palm
b) Partial thickness (second degree) burns are typically painless and insensate
c) In the "rule of 9's" the % body surface area of a whole leg equates to 18%
d) Superficial (first degree) burns frequently require skin grafting
e) In the acute setting, partial and full thickness burns are easily discernable

[Best Answer = c]

Explanation

The size of the patients palm (not the clinicians) approximates to 1% of their BSA. Partial thickness burns are painful, erythematous, mottled and associated with swelling and blisters. Superficial burns (first degree) cause erythema and cytokine release, and heal well without scarring. Differentiating between partial and full thickness burns is difficult in the acute setting and advice should be taken where uncertainty exists.

11. Regarding abdominal trauma in an unconscious patient

a) The diaphragm reaches xiphisternal level during inspiration
b) A laparotomy is indicated for blunt injuries
c) Major injuries can be reliably excluded by careful abdominal examination
d) Failure to respond to fluid resuscitation mandates an urgent CT scan
e) Diagnostic peritoneal lavage (DPL) is highly sensitive for intraperitoneal bleeding

[Best Answer = e]

Explanation

During expiration the diaphragm can reach nipple level. This is important to consider when dealing with penetrating injuries to the lower chest and so an intra-abdominal injury cannot be ruled out. In addition, the trajectory of the instrument may damage below the level of the entry point. In general blunt trauma should be managed conservatively where at all possible although clinical examination is not always reliable. Failure to respond to fluid resuscitation in a patient suspected of having abdominal trauma indicates the need for urgent surgery. An unstable patient should not be transferred into a potentially dangerous environment for a CT scan.

12. With regard to pelvic fractures

a) Pelvic X-rays should be taken in all patients with multi-system trauma
b) Digital rectal examination is diagnostic
c) Urethral catheterisation should be performed as soon as urethral injury is suspected
d) Shenton's lines are always disrupted
e) Shock is common in isolated pubic rami fractures

[Best Answer = a]

Explanation

The pelvic X-ray is taken as part of the initial trauma series along with the chest and lateral c-spine. Digital rectal examination is important in identifying rectal injuries, a "high riding" prostate and diminished anal tone. A palpable sharp bone end should also increase your index of suspicion although a normal rectal examination clearly cannot rule out a pelvic fracture. If urethral trauma is suspected, a urethral catheter should not be inserted until a urethrogram is performed. Shenton's line is an imaginary line that follows the inferior margin of the neck of femur which continues with the superior margin of the obturator foramen. In certain pelvic fractures, such as those of the superior pubic ramus, Shenton's line can be disrupted. Usually, disruption of Shenton's line or asymmetry between sides is a sign of a fractured neck of the femur. Isolated pubic rami fractures are not usually associated with major haemorrhage.

13. Shock

a) Blood pressure is maintained in stage 3 shock
b) Neurogenic shock results in vasoconstriction
c) Systemic vascular resistance increases with anaphylactic shock
d) Cardiogenic shock may occur secondary to an arrhythmia
e) Thirty per cent blood loss equates to around 500 ml in a 70 kg adult

[Best Answer = d]

Explanation

Blood pressure falls in grade 3 shock, since the blood loss exceeds 30%. In neurogenic shock (where there is spinal transection) there is a loss of sympathetic outflow below the lesion, resulting in vasodilatation. Anaphylatic shock causes vasodilatation resulting in reduced systemic vascular resistance. Causes of primary cardiogenic shock include myocardial infarction, arrhythmia, and valvular heart disease. The normal circulating volume in an adult is 70 ml/kg which is approximately 5000 ml in a 70 kg man and hence 30% is approximately 1.5 L.

14. Burns

a) Arsenic poisoning should commonly be considered in house fires
b) In the Muir-Barclay formula the fluid volume is proportional to the patient's age
c) Tetanus immunisation must be given
d) IV cannulae for fluid resuscitation should never be placed through burned skin
e) Are a major cause of fatal accidents in children

[Best Answer = e]

Explanation

Burning plastic can cause hydrogen cyanide (not arsenic) poisoning which is particularly a problem with old style foam-filled furniture. Fluid requirements from the Muir-Barclay formula are the product of

(% Burn × Weight in kg) / 2. Whenever tetanus immunisation status is uncertain appropriate vaccination should be given. Burns covering >20% BSA require circulating volume support. Overlying burned skin is not a contraindication to IV cannula placement if lines cannot be established in unburned skin.

15. Central line insertion

a) The Seldinger technique is contraindicated
b) Head down tilt reduces the risk of air embolism
c) A chest X-ray is unnecessary post-procedure
d) In the mid internal jugular approach the cannula is aimed at the contralateral nipple
e) The subclavian vein is deep to the artery below the clavicle

[Best Answer = b]

Explanation

The Seldinger technique is the standard method for inserting central lines both in the subclavian and internal jugular approaches. Head down tilt reduces the risk of air embolus and distends the neck veins. A post-procedure X-ray is essential to check the line positioning and to rule out complications (pneumothorax and haemothorax). In the internal jugular approach, the cannula should be directed towards the ipsilateral nipple. The subclavian vein is superficial to the artery.

Case Studies

Case 1

Whilst out running a 25-year-old male is hit on his left side by a van travelling at 20 mph. On arrival of the ambulance he is alert, orientated and moving all his limbs. His heart rate and BP are 76 bpm and 116/70 mmHg, respectively. During transfer to hospital, venous access is obtained with a 14G cannula in his left ante-cubital fossa, through which 1000 ml of crystalloid is given. When he arrives at A&E his observations are 93 bpm & 117/90 mmHg.

a) How should oxygen therapy be administered?

b) Is venous access appropriate?

c) Comment on his vital signs.

d) What life-threatening chest injuries should be focused on in the primary survey?

e) The chest X-ray demonstrates fractures of the left ninth and tenth ribs later-ally and blunting of the left costophrenic angle. What abdominal injury would you be suspicious of?

Answers

> a) High flow oxygen should be delivered via a face mask with a reservoir bag to all trauma patients.
>
> b) The location and size of the existing IV cannula is correct, but trauma patients should always have a minimum of two large bore cannulae.
>
> c) His initial observations are acceptable, however, it is worth considering that fit patients compensate considerably for blood loss and his normal resting heart rate may be less than 60. Absolute vital sign measurements are important but so is their trend especially in response to treatment. In this case the patient's heart rate has increased despite 1000 ml of fluid. His systolic BP has not changed but his pulse pressure has decreased which suggests an increase in circulating catecholamines, and peripheral vascular resistance. A chest injury or intra-abdominal bleeding should be seriously considered.

Case 2

A 60-year-old lady with long standing COPD escaped from a house fire where an electric heater set fire to her bedroom furniture. She sustained partial thickness burns to the anterior aspect of both legs, thighs and right upper limb. Although there were no obvious burns to her face and her voice was audible she was continually coughing.

a) What is the first priority?
b) What signs might suggest an inhalation injury?
c) When should the anaesthetic team be involved?
d) What other investigations should be done at this stage?
e) What general management steps are required in this burns patient?

Answers

a) High flow humidified oxygen should be given immediately. If the patient has a patent airway she should be sat up in a comfortable position. This will reduce airway oedema and improve ventilatory function. Do not attempt to insert any airway devices until help has arrived, unless absolutely necessary, for fear of causing further distress to the patient.
b) Obvious signs include stridor and hoarseness, but more subtle signs include facial burns, singed eyebrows or nasal hair, carbonaceous sputum, and drooling/wheeze.
c) The anaesthetic team should be warned as soon as possible given a history suggestive of possible inhalation injury as the supra-glottic airway can rapidly become obstructed due to oedema.
d) An arterial blood gas, CO-haemoglobin levels, and CXR are important initially. Note pulse oximetry is of limited value as it

cannot differentiate between oxy-haemoglobin and CO-haemo-globin and thus gives falsely high values.

e) Appropriate fluid resuscitation, assessment of burn depth and surface area affected, as well as identifying associated injuries and analgesia requirements.

Case 3

A young security guard sustained a stab would to the right side of his chest with a sharp object and was promptly driven to A&E by a colleague. Despite initially appearing well on arrival to A&E he was gasping for breath. The nursing staff immediately gave him high flow oxygen and connected him to monitoring — ECG, BP, HR, SpO₂, and RR.

a) You arrive on scene; the patient is obviously extremely unwell, what are your initial actions?

b) With tracheal deviation away from the site of injury, and a stab wound to the right eighth intercostal space what is the most likely diagnosis and what do you do?

After an initial improvement in his condition, it is now noted that the patient has become clammy and irritable. His heart rate has increased to 120 although his blood pressure is around the normal range.

c) In view of his deterioration what should be suspected?

d) How can this be confirmed?

Answers

a) Call for help; primary survey; adequate IV access; simultaneously treat problems that are identified in the ABC of the primary survey.

b) The clinical situation fits with a tension pneumothorax. This is a clinical diagnosis, and if suspected should initially be treated with an urgent needle decompression. Do not wait for a CXR to confirm your suspicion!

c) Assuming the chest drain is swinging satisfactory and the CXR post-drain insertion showed no other injuries and a good drain position, then concealed haemorrhage into the abdomen should always be at the back of your mind, when dealing with penetrating injuries to the lower chest.

Correct functioning of the chest drain can be checked either by looking for swinging of the fluid level with breathing or asking the patient to cough to see bubbles escaping. When abdominal trauma is considered there is a choice of investigations: Diagnostic Peritoneal Lavage (DPL), CT scanning and Ultrasound (USS). The choice of investigation should involve a senior clinician and will depend on the stability of the patient and in some centres the accessibility of the particular investigation. DPL — Is rapid, safe, and sensitive for the presence of intraperitoneal blood, but does not identify source of bleeding. It can also miss retroperitoneal injuries and is an invasive procedure. CT — Assists in managing certain types of injury conservatively, and identifies some injuries missed by DPL. In most hospitals CT scanning involves moving a potentially unstable patient into an isolated environment, which can be dangerous. USS — Portable, rapid (when available in close proximity), non-invasive, and accurate for significant haemorrhage. However USS requires skill to use, and cannot always identify all organs clearly and the source of the problem precisely.

Case 4

A 60-year-old man with chronic alcohol dependence falls down and bangs his head outside a social club after a "good" night out. Although he is alert and orientated a passerby calls for an ambulance as the patient is known to live alone. On arrival at hospital he is noted to have a mild occipital contusion. Neurological examination is unremarkable other than some mild ataxia.

a) What features in his social history are pertinent in his management?
b) Will a skull X-ray aid your management?
c) What observations should a "head injuries" (neurological observations) chart include?
d) What are the signs to look out for in a base of skull fracture?
e) What type of cerebral injury are chronic alcoholics at increased risk of, and what vessels are usually responsible?

Answers

a) Patients with chronic alcohol intake are at increased incidence of significant head injury. Alcohol intoxication makes assessment of the patient more difficult; but bear in mind that neurological findings cannot be assumed to be secondary to alcohol intake.

b) The presence of a skull fracture will indicate that the patient is at increased risk of a significant cerebral injury, but its absence alone cannot disprove a significant head injury. (Note: In a fully conscious patient the risk of an intracranial haematoma is 1:30 in the presence of a skull fracture and <1:1000 without a fracture).

c) Glasgow Coma Scale (GCS); pupilary response and size; limb movement; HR; BP; temperature; and respiratory rate should be recorded.

d) Signs of base of skull fracture include: CSF otorrhoea; CSF rhinorrhoea; haemotympanum; "Panda eyes" (bruising confined to the orbital margins); and "Battle's sign" (bruising over the mastoid process).

e) Patients with a history of chronic alcohol abuse develop cerebral atrophy and are at risk of subdural haemorrhage due to tearing of the cortical bridging veins.

Case 5

A 40-year-old engineer was electrocuted whilst working at an electrical substation. Contact was made between his right arm and the positive AC electrical supply.

a) In the absence of vital signs, what is the treatment of an electrocution victim?
b) What feature of the domestic electrical supply makes it particularly hazardous?
c) Why are electrical burns so damaging to tissues?
d) What is the significance of entry and exit sites?
e) What complications can occur secondary to muscle necrosis?
f) What syndrome is he at risk of with a muscle injury to his limb?

Answers

a) Cardiopulmonary resuscitation should be instituted along national guidelines (assumes the environment is now safe).

b) The frequency of current in a domestic electrical supply is 50 Hz. This frequency has a high risk of inducing ventricular fibrillation.

c) Electrical current will follow the routes of least resistance through the tissues. Nerves, blood vessels, and muscle are at particularly affected as they offer the least resistance to current flow. Injury is caused by direct heat and subsequent necrosis and thrombosis.

d) If electricity has passed through the patient there are usually two or more entry / exit wounds. Full thickness burns with a charred white edge suggest internal damage from an electrical burn. The internal damage (such as muscle necrosis) may far exceed the limited external appearance.

e) Muscle necrosis leads to myoglobin release, hyperkalaemia, and acidosis. Myoglobin release from damaged muscle cells can induce acute renal failure, hence adequate hydration and a good urine output should be maintained.

f) Electrical damage to muscle causes swelling and thereby increases the compartment pressure compromising tissue perfusion. All such patients must have careful circulatory observations to watch for the development of compartment syndrome.

Extended Matching Questions

EMQ 1

a. Tension pneumothorax
b. Pelvic fracture
c. Cardiac tamponade
d. Airway obstruction
e. Uncomplicated pneumothorax
f. Haemothorax
g. Aortic disruption
h. Flail chest injury

Choose a diagnosis from the list above, which most fits the trauma case scenarios described below:

1) Shock associated with absent breath sounds / dull percussion note of right lung field.
2) Injury to the chest with paradoxical motion of chest wall and hyperventilation.
3) Fractured left sided ribs after a fall, respiratory distress and trachea displaced towards the right.
4) Penetrating chest trauma; muffled heart sounds; jugular venous distension; and decreased BP.
5) Widened mediastinum.

Answers

> **1) f.**
> Dull percussion note to the chest with absent breath sounds would suggest fluid within the chest. In a shocked trauma patient, the most likely diagnosis would be a large haemothorax.
>
> **2) h.**
> Paradoxical moment of the chest wall suggests a chest wall injury with a flail segment.
>
> **3) a.**
> Respiratory distress and displacement of the trachea away from the injury suggest a tension pneumothorax. In addition you would expect absent breath sounds and a hyper-resonant chest on the affected side.

4) c.

Beck's triad consisting of increased central venous pressure, decreased blood pressure and muffled heart sounds are features of a cardiac tamponade. In reality, muffled heart sounds may be difficult to ascertain in a noisy trauma environment. In the trauma situation the key to correct diagnosis is having a high index of suspicion with the mechanism of injury, e.g. steering wheel trauma or chest stab wound.

5) g.

The patient reaching A&E with a disruption of the thoracic aorta will have a contained leak, free ruptures will have died on scene. There are a variety of other X-ray signs described, but a widened mediastinum is probably the easiest to appreciate.

EMQ 2

a. Pelvic fracture
b. Spinal injury
c. Urethral injury
d. Sternal fracture
e. Fractured neck of femur
f. Pneumothorax
g. Testicular torsion
h. Splenic rupture
i. Fracture to the femoral shaft
j. Microscopic haematuria

Select the most appropriate option for the patients described below:

1) Fall from a horse in a 25-year-old lady who has hypotension that responds to fluid resuscitation. She has a normal CXR. The abdominal USS shows minimal fluid in the abdomen and there is no evidence of long bone fracture.
2) A 70-year-old driver involved in a head-on collision with a wall at 30 mph. ECG demonstrated ST elevation in anterior leads and there is evidence of patchy pulmonary opacification.
3) A 30-year-old rugby player kicked in his flank. He is stable and has normal vital signs.
4) A 60-year-old man knocked down by a car. His right leg is shortened with swelling and deformity of the thigh. No other injuries are found and he is tachycardic on arrival.

5) A 35-year-old motorcyclist knocked off his bike at 50 mph. No evidence of long bone deformity. He has hypotension with bradycardia and paralysis of the legs.

Answers

1) a.
Hypotension that has responded to fluid resuscitation would suggest contained bleeding. Pelvic fractures should be considered in such a fall, particularly when other sources of blood loss are not apparent.

2) d.
Sternal fractures often occur in RTA's related to a seat belt injury or impact with the steering wheel. When severe they can be associated with pulmonary and cardiac contusion. Sternal fractures are best seen on a lateral sternal X-ray.

3) j.
Microscopic haematuria is not an uncommon finding in contact sports where blows occur to the loin. In the majority of cases there is no significant underlying renal injury.

4) i.
The location of a femoral fracture affects the limbs position. In a femoral shaft fracture there may be shortening of the leg, abduction at the hip, external rotation of the leg and thigh swelling. In addition haemorrhagic complications are greater from femoral shaft compared with femoral neck fractures.

5) b.
Spinal injuries should be suspected in trauma victims in the presence of any of the following: diaphragmatic breathing; hypotension with bradycardia (spinal shock); decreased anal tone; loss of sensation below the clavicles; and paralysis.

EMQ 3

a. CO level of 33%
b. Second degree burns to both legs and anterior abdominal wall
c. Extrication from house fire
d. Forty per cent superficial (first degree) burns
e. High-tension electrocution with entry and exit wound

f. Circumferential full thickness burns to forearm
g. Chemical burn with cement
h. Oxygen saturations of 85%
i. Paediatric non-accidental injury
j. Explosion from gas canister

Select the most appropriate scenario for the patients described below:

1) A patient requiring escharotomy.
2) An injury requiring copious washing with water.
3) A patient to be considered for hyperbaric O_2 therapy.
4) A patient with myoglobinuria.
5) A patient with a liver laceration.

Answers

1) f.
Circumferential full thickness burns to the forearm may compromise its viability and require fasciotomies to decompress the distal limb.

2) g.
Washing with copious amounts of water is particularly important in the case of chemical burns.

3) a.
Hyperbaric oxygen therapy should be considered in patients with CO levels >30%.

4) e.
Myoglobin release signifies muscle damage.

5) j.
Patients with burns involved in blast injuries and forceful accidents should be considered at high risk of other injuries such as blunt abdominal and chest trauma.

EMQ 4

a. CSF rhinorrhoea
b. Berry aneurysm
c. Childhood history of seizures

d. VII cranial nerve palsy
e. Severe acceleration / deceleration injury
f. Major blood loss
g. Treatment with warfarin
h. Whiplash
i. Lucid interval

Select the feature above most consistent with the following head injuries:

1) Base of skull fracture.
2) Extensive scalp laceration.
3) Extradural haemorrhage.
4) Subdural haemorrhage.
5) Diffuse axonal injury.

Answers

1) a.
CSF rhinorrhoea is leakage of CSF from the nose. It is a feature of a base of skull fracture as is Battle's sign, which is bruising over the mastoid.

2) f.
Do not underestimate the amount of blood loss from scalp lacerations, which can be major.

3) i.
Damage to the middle meningeal artery from fractures of the temporal bone is the usual cause of extradural haemorrhage. There is typically a loss of consciousness immediately post-head injury, and a return to full consciousness (lucid interval) before the neurological deterioration occurs as the haematoma develops.

4) g.
Patients on warfarin therapy are more prone to subdural haemorrhage following head injuries.

5) e.
Diffuse axonal injury results from shearing forces within the brain tissue from acceleration/deceleration injuries. It frequently has a poor prognosis and is often difficult to differentiate from hypoxic brain injury.

EMQ 5

a. High central venous pressure and low cardiac output
b. Hypercalcaemia
c. Urticaria and bronchospasm
d. Loss of sympathetic tone
e. Severe burns
f. Intracranial haematoma
g. Paracetamol overdose
h. Hypoglycaemia
i. Sinus arrhythmia
j. Fever and vasodilatation

Select the features/diagnosis most consistent with the following:

1) Neurogenic shock.
2) Anaphylactic shock.
3) Cardiogenic shock.
4) Hypovolaemic shock.
5) Septic shock.

Answers

1) d.
Neurogenic shock results from damage to the sympathetic pathways of the spinal cord. This causes loss of vasomotor tone and hypotension. In a multiple injured trauma patient this can exacerbate the physiological effects of hypovolaemia.

2) c.
Anaphylactic shock occurs as a result of immunological responses following exposure to a trigger agent. Typically the patient has angio-oedema, urticaria, dyspnoea and hypotension. Cardiovascular collapse occurs secondary to vasodilatation and loss of plasma from the circulating compartment. Bronchospasm is present in 50% of cases.

3) a.
Cardiogenic shock is caused by pump failure, which physiologically is reflected by a low cardiac output, increased filling pressures (CVP) and increased systemic vascular resistance.

4) e.

Hypovolaemic shock results as a loss of circulating volume (low CVP and BP). This can be due to loss of blood, plasma (as in major burns), or extravascular fluid (e.g. dehydration).

5) j.

Septic shock results in inadequate tissue perfusion caused by an infective agent. Inflammatory mediators are triggered which cause systemic effects such as increased capillary permeability, fever, and vasodilatation.

Chapter 2   Liver, Biliary Tract and Pancreas

Rajiv Lochan and Richard Charnley

Multiple Choice Questions

[Each single best answer (SBA) question comprises a stem and a number of answers. You are asked to decide which single item represents the best answer to the question.]

1. **Obstructive jaundice is not caused by**

    a) Bile duct stones
    b) Viral hepatitis
    c) Tumours of the pancreas
    d) Duodenal tumours
    e) Enlarged lymph nodes at the porta hepatis

[Best Answer = b]

Explanation

Obstructive jaundice can occur due to bile duct stones and tumours of the head of pancreas and biliary tract. Duodenal and pyloric tumours can also cause obstructive jaundice by directly involving the bile duct or by metastasising to the lymph nodes around the duct and the porta where they can cause obstruction (mainly in stomach neoplasms/ lymphomas). Severe viral hepatitis can cause a mixed hepatocellular/ cholestatic picture of LFTs but the clinical picture and the severe elevation of transaminases should make the distinction straightforward. Drugs can also sometimes cause a cholestatic elevation in LFTs but they are also not causes of obstructive jaundice.

2. **Obstructive jaundice due to carcinoma of the pancreas is not usually associated with**

    a) Yellow colouration of skin and mucous membranes
    b) Itching
    c) Dark coloured urine

d) Pale clay-like stools

e) Abdominal pain

[Best Answer = e]

Explanation

Depending on the cause, jaundice can be associated with various other symptoms. Obstruction to the outflow of bile from the liver results in the absence of bile in the gut leading to pale, clay-like stools. Dark urine ("tea" or "cola" coloured urine) results from excretion of conjugated bilirubin, which occurs in obstructive jaundice. Itching results from the deposition of bile salts in the dermis. Abdominal pain with or without fever suggests an underlying inflammatory or infective pathology. Painless jaundice is often an indicator of a neoplastic cause.

3. **In a patient with jaundice, your first investigation would be:**

a) ERCP

b) Liver function tests and abdominal ultrasound

c) CT scan

d) Laparoscopy

e) MRCP (magnetic resonance cholangio-pancreatography)

[Best Answer = b]

Explanation

After a history and clinical examination, your first line investigations would be liver function tests and an ultrasound scan (USS) of the liver and biliary tract. The results of which will guide further investigation in a patient with jaundice. A predominant elevation of transaminases amongst the liver enzymes along with normal bile ducts on the USS will suggest a medical cause for the jaundice such as viral hepatitis. Elevated alkaline phosphatase and/or γ-glutamyl transferase levels and dilatation of the whole or a portion of the biliary tract will indicate a surgical cause for the jaundice. Axial imaging such as computed tomography and or MRI/MRCP are further tests which may be needed. ERCP is invasive and is not a first-line test.

4. **The following may be indications for the performance of ERCP**

   a) Diagnosis of a bile duct calculus
   b) Removal of a bile duct calculus
   c) Assessment of biliary stent patency
   d) Diagnosis of pancreas divisum
   e) Diagnosis of chronic pancreatitis

[Best Answer = b]

Explanation

Endoscopic retrograde cholangio-pancreatography is an invasive procedure which is, with a few exceptions, reserved for therapeutic procedures such as known bile duct stones, lower biliary stricture requiring drainage and complications of chronic pancreatitis requiring stenting or stone extraction. This is because of the significant complications (8%–10% morbidity and 0.3%–1% procedure related mortality) associated with it. These include acute pancreatitis, bleeding (from the site of sphincterotomy), biliary infection and perforation of the duodenum. High definition imaging modalities such as magnetic resonance cholangio-pancreatography (MRCP) (for the diagnosis of pancreas divisum and CBD stones), endoscopic ultrasound (for bile duct stones, chronic pancreatitis and pancreatic and periampullary tumours) and thin-slice CT (for pancreatic masses) are preferred to invasive modalities like ERCP. ERCP should therefore be reserved for therapy.

5. **Ultrasound scanning is poor at identifying the following in a patient with obstructive jaundice**

   a) Dilated intra-hepatic ducts
   b) Dilated extra-hepatic ducts
   c) Gall bladder stones

d) Pancreatic masses

e) Intra-hepatic masses

[Best Answer = d]

Explanation

> Ultrasound scanning uses sound waves to image the internal struc-
> tures of an organ. Although reliable in the identification of gall blad-
> der stones, biliary dilatation and liver tumours, 80%–90% of patients
> with CBD stones and 50% of patients with pancreatic tumours remain
> undiagnosed following abdominal ultrasound. This is because there is
> significant interference due to the presence of gas-filled bowel loops
> in the vicinity of the lower bile duct.

6. **Which of the following is not part of the pre-op preparation of a deeply
   jaundiced patient for ERCP?**

   a) Adequate hydration (overnight maintenance IV fluids)
   b) Check and confirm normal coagulation parameters
   c) Prophylactic antibiotics
   d) Informed consent
   e) Oral vitamin "K"

[Best Answer = e]

Explanation

> Adequate hydration of jaundiced patients is essential because renal
> impairment can easily occur in these patients, especially when they
> are being fasted on multiple occasions for various procedures during
> their hospital stay. Obstructive jaundice results in impaired absorp-
> tion of fat soluble vitamins including vitamin "K" which can lead to
> impaired coagulation reliably corrected by parenteral not oral vitamin
> "K". Impaired coagulation must be corrected before intervention
> since these procedures are associated with a significant incidence of
> bleeding. Instrumentation of the biliary tract is associated with a high
> incidence of biliary sepsis, which can easily result in septicaemia.

7. **Which of the following is not a cause of acute pancreatitis?**

a) Trauma
b) ERCP
c) Bile duct stones
d) Hypomagnaesemia
e) Mutations in the cystic fibrosis transmembrane regulator gene

[Best Answer = d]

Explanation

In the UK, nearly 60% of all cases of acute pancreatitis are caused by biliary calculi and 20% by alcohol. Bouts of excessive consumption (binge drinking) are often responsible. ERCP is thought to be responsible for about 4%–5% of cases. Trauma, drugs and infections (mainly viral e.g. mumps) are each responsible for about 1%–2%, biochemical abnormalities such as hypercalcaemia and hypertriglyceridaemia each for about 2%–4%. Genetic abnormalities such as mutations of the CFTR gene and hereditary pancreatitis (secondary to mutations in the cationic trypsinogen gene) cause 2%–3% of cases and it is likely that this cohort of patients will be increasingly identifiable in the future with many more genetic abnormalities being recognised. Ten per cent of cases are presently labelled as idiopathic. Hypomagnaesemia might be a result of malabsorption but is not a known cause of pancreatitis. The mnemonic GET SMASH'N is often used by students — gallstones, ethanol, trauma, steroids (and other drugs including asathioprine), mumps (and other viral infections including coxsackie B), autoimmune diseases (e.g. SLE), scorpion bites (rare and not in the UK), hyperlipidaemia (and hyperparathyroidism, hypothermia and hereditary causes) and neoplasia.

8. **Which of the following are not indicated in the initial management of a patient with acute pancreatitis?**

a) Resuscitation with intravenous fluids and maintenance of intra-vascular volume
b) Urgent CT scan of the abdomen
c) Close monitoring of urine output

d) Pain relief

e) Arterial blood gases

[Best Answer = b]

Explanation

The initial manifestation and early complications of acute pancreatitis are due to a massive systemic inflammatory response (SIRS) which results in "leaky capillaries". This causes significant fluid and electrolyte losses into the "third space" — which is not visible or quantifiable externally. The identification and correction of this is the most important initial phase of management. The micro-circulation in the lung is extremely sensitive to SIRS and this is the first organ to decompensate following acute pancreatitis and hence close attention to respiratory status is important. Intravenous antibiotics do not prevent the development of pancreatic necrosis. Prophylactic antibiotics are only indicated in predicted severe acute pancreatitis and only for seven days unless a positive culture is obtained. A contrast CT within the first three days is not indicated but in severe cases a CT three to ten days after the onset of the attack is useful to diagnose necrosis if present. Enteral nutrition as soon as ileus settles has been proven to be of benefit in acute pancreatitis. TPN is indicated following the initial resuscitation only if enteral feeding is contraindicated.

9. **Which of the following would not normally be carried out in an outpatient setting, for a patient who was discharged three weeks ago following an apparently idiopathic attack of mild acute pancreatitis?**

a) Take a detailed family history

b) Estimate serum lipids

c) Check serum calcium

d) Repeat the Ultrasound scan of the abdomen

e) ERCP

[Best Answer = e]

Explanation

> The common and easily identifiable causes should be investigated initially and this is done by a detailed life-style and family history. Past history of abdominal trauma should be specifically looked for. Evidence of biliary calculi and biochemical abnormalities are easily documented with simple investigations — blood tests and ultrasonography of the biliary tract. Hypercalcaemia is a known cause of pancreatitis). An ERCP or CT scan is not initially indicated following a complete recovery from acute pancreatitis.

10. Which of the following are not independent risk factors for pancreatic cancer?

a) Increasing age
b) Tobacco smoking
c) Coffee consumption
d) Chronic pancreatitis
e) Hereditary non-polyposis colorectal cancer (HNPCC)

[Best Answer = c]

Explanation

> Increasing age, male gender and tobacco smoking are strong risk factors for pancreatic cancer. Hereditary non-polyposis colorectal cancer is an autosomal dominantly inherited disorder of DNA mismatch repair proteins in which colorectal cancers occur. This syndrome is responsible for about 5% of hereditary pancreatic cancers. Ten percent of all cases of pancreatic cancer are thought to have a hereditary basis. Consumption of coffee has been disproven to play a role in cancer of the pancreas. Alcohol consumption by itself is not an independent risk factor although chronic pancreatitis is responsible for about 5%–10% of cases of pancreatic cancer. However, the development of malignancy in a chronically inflamed pancreas is exceedingly difficult to prove.

11. Which of the following is not a complication of biliary calculi?

a) Acute cholecystitis
b) Empyema of gall bladder
c) Liver abscesses
d) Chronic hepatitis
e) Acute cholangitis

[Best Answer = d]

Explanation

Gall bladder calculi can cause acute or recurrent chronic inflammation of the gall bladder and hence cholecystitis. They can cause a complete obstruction to the neck of the gall bladder and the resulting bacterial infection can cause an empyema ("collection of pus within a natural body cavity") of the gall bladder. Calculi within the bile ducts can do the same and result in acute cholangitis. Ascending infection results in seeding of the liver and subsequent abscess formation. Chronic hepatitis is not a result of biliary calculi.

12. Which of the following are not associated with the aetiology of chronic pancreatitis?

a) Alcohol abuse
b) Tobacco smoking
c) Tropical pancreatitis
d) Autoimmunity
e) A positive family history

[Best Answer = b]

Explanation

Acute biliary pancreatitis usually does not progress to chronic pancreatitis unlike alcohol induced pancreatitis. Microlithiasis of the biliary tract however is thought to cause chronic pancreatitis by repeated subclinical inflammation of the pancreas. Apart from alcohol the other major cause of chronic pancreatitis is genetic mutations which include mutations of the cationic trypsinogen gene (causing hereditary pancreatitis) and CFTR gene. Tropical pancreatitis is a type of chronic inflammation found in Southern India, the aetiology of which is unclear. Tobacco smoking by itself is not a causative factor, but plays an additive role.

13. The following are true of liver abscesses

a) A viral source of infection should be looked for
b) Pyogenic abscesses are often caused by staphlococcus epidermidis
c) Open operation is invariable
d) Colonic tumours can occasionally present as liver abscesses
e) Amoebiasis is the most common cause of liver abscess in the UK

[Best Answer = d]

Explanation

Liver abscess are usually secondary to a bacterial infection in the peritoneal cavity, most usually the colon (diverticulitis), appendicitis or biliary sepsis and hence an intra-abdominal source of infection should be looked for. When the biliary tree is the source of infection enteric Gram-negative aerobic Bacilli and Enterococci are common isolates. In a significant proportion of cases the primary cause is not found and these are usually colonised by *Streptococcus mileri*. Although Staphylococcus can be a cause (especially in those where haematogenous spread is the cause) this is in fact rare. Primary amoebic liver abscesses are rare in the Western world, but common in the Middle-East, Southern and Eastern parts of Asia and Africa. Percutaneous drainage is the first line of treatment, but open drainage or liver resection may be necessary in selected cases. Colonic tumours can present as an abscess in the liver.

14. Pancreatic tumours

a) Are usually associated with abdominal pain at an early stage
b) Acinar cell carcinoma is the most common histological type

c) Metastases to the pancreas are likely to be from the kidney or breast
d) Tumours in the body and tail are more common than those situated in the head of the organ
e) Chemotherapy is effective

[Best Answer = c]

Explanation

The presentation of pancreatic neoplasms depends upon their anatomical situation. Tumours in the head of the pancreas classically present with painless obstructive jaundice and are more common (60%–70% of all cases) than those arising within the body/tail of the organ, which present in an advanced state usually with backache and weight loss. Metastasis to the pancreas is uncommon, but is usually from a primary in the kidney or breast. Ductal adenocarcinoma is the most common histological type of pancreatic cancer. The others are rare and are: acinar cell carcinoma, adenosquamous carcinoma, various cystic tumours and neuro-endocrine neoplasms. Chemotherapy by itself is not very effective, but recent trials have demonstrated a survival benefit for patients who have received adjuvant chemotherapy following a successful resection of the primary pancreatic neoplasm.

15. Liver tumours

a) Are usually primary neoplasms
b) Hepatocellular carcinoma (HCC) is rarely associated with cirrhosis
c) Usually present with severe derangement of liver function tests
d) Are usually symptomatic
e) Surgical removal of metastases from colo-rectal tumours is accepted treatment for solitary tumours

[Best Answer = e]

Explanation

Most malignant neoplasms of the liver are metastases, mainly from the lung, breast, colon or pancreas. Resection of liver metastases from a previous colorectal primary is accepted treatment for solitary metastases and selected patients with multiple metastases. However these patients have to be carefully staged and surgery forms a part of multidisciplinary treatment. Hepatocellular carcinoma is the most common primary liver neoplasm and commonly occurs in a cirrhotic liver, though the fibro lamellar variety which is more common in young/middle females occurs in a normal liver and is associated with a better prognosis. Most liver masses can be asymptomatic for a long time and severe derangement of liver function is unusual except in the case of HCC occurring in a cirrhotic liver.

Case Studies

Case 1

A 55-year-old woman presents with a three-day history of upper abdominal pain radiating through to the region of her right scapula, which was intermittent initially, but has been constant for the past day. On examination she is febrile and has tenderness and guarding in the RUQ.

a) What is your clinical diagnosis?
b) What is the clinical sign which is usually thought to clinch the diagnosis?
c) How will you investigate this patient?
d) What is the confirmatory investigation?
e) What are the initial steps in the management?
f) What complications will you expect and look out for?
g) What is the definitive treatment option?

Answers

a) The most likely diagnosis would be acute cholecystitis. The initial intermittent nature of the pain would be compatible with biliary colic. As the gall bladder becomes progressively obstructed, inflammation occurs resulting in constant pain. Associated pyrexia indicates the likelihood of bacterial infection.

b) A positive Murphy's sign is the clinching clinical finding. This is elicited by applying gentle pressure in the right hypochondrium with the flat of the right hand and asking the patient to breathe in deeply. A positive sign causes the patient to catch his/her breath due to irritation of the peritoneum lining the exterior of the gall bladder. Eliciting this sign results in great discomfort to the patient.

c) Routine investigations would include FBC, LFTs, U + Es and serum amylase. Some abnormalities of LFTs are seen in 20% of patients mainly as raised alkaline phosphatase with or without raised bilirubin levels.

d) An ultrasound scan of the abdomen may demonstrate oedema and thickening of the gall bladder wall associated with the presence of peri-cholecystic fluid. Gall bladder stones are visualised in 90% of patients.

e) Initial treatment is conservative — pain relief with opiates, I.V. rehydration and antibiotics — usually a broad spectrum cephalosporin in combination with metronidazole. Patients are restricted to clear fluids for the initial one to two days. About 10% of patients do not settle with this treatment and will need early cholecystectomy.

f) The complications which can occur with acute cholecystitis are cholangitis, acute pancreatitis, empyema of the gall bladder, gangrenous cholecystitis, Mirizzi syndrome and chronic cholecystitis.

g) The definitive treatment in patients who settle with conservative treatment is laparoscopic cholecystectomy which is usually performed six to eight weeks following the acute episode. Immediate surgery, however, is gaining in popularity and is as safe as delayed surgery.

Case 2

A 35-year-old male is brought to the A&E by the ambulance crew, who were called to his house by his wife. She reports that he was well six hours previously when he complained of sudden onset of severe upper abdominal pain radiating to the back. He subsequently started vomiting and has become progressively unwell. On examination he is conscious but severely dehydrated and shocked with a pulse of 120 beats per minute, BP 80/40, RR 26, SaO$_2$ 94% (room air). He has severe upper abdominal tenderness and guarding with no masses.

a) What are your initial steps in the management of this patient?
b) What are the differential diagnoses you would entertain and what investigations will you request?
c) If this patient was diagnosed with acute pancreatitis what will be your next step?
d) What investigations will this patient need once he is stable?
e) How will you predict the severity of an attack of acute pancreatitis?
f) What are the complications of acute pancreatitis?

Answers

a) The priority is to resuscitate this patient. Assess airway breathing and circulation. The essentials are to achieve good secure venous access, send peripheral blood off for investigations and commence resuscitation with boluses of crystalloids. Supplemental oxygen is essential. Adequacy of resuscitation is assessed by estimating tissue or end organ perfusion. A urinary catheter to monitor urine output is essential. If haemodynamics do not improve with two to four litres of fluid replacement an intensivist should be involved, sooner rather than later.

b) The differential diagnoses are acute pancreatitis, hollow viscus perforation, myocardial infarction, a dissecting aortic aneurysm and acute mesenteric ischaemia. The investigations (in addition to routine haematology and blood biochemistry) which will help in this situation are serum amylase, ECG, erect chest X-ray and an urgent contrast CT. A serum amylase level of three to four times more than the upper limit of normal laboratory value will confirm the diagnosis of acute pancreatitis in this setting. Free air under the diaphragm makes the diagnosis of perforated hollow viscous in 70% of cases. In a clinical situation where you very strongly suspect this and an erect CXR is normal, a CT scan will make the diagnosis. Acute MI can be diagnosed with its classical changes on an ECG, and elevated troponin "T" levels, however various ECG changes can occur in acute pancreatitis and an MI can occur in patients who have suffered an acute attack of pancreatitis. Most major vascular catastrophes can be diagnosed on a contrast CT scan.

c) Following adequate resuscitation, including transfer to an intensive care/high dependency unit, the next step will be to assess severity of the episode of pancreatitis and to ascertain the cause of the attack.

d) An urgent ultrasound scan within 24 hours of admission is indicated. This is because urgent ERCP is beneficial in severe acute biliary pancreatitis.

e) The level of elevation of the serum amylase does not correlate with severity of the attack. Individual patient factors and biochemical measurements have been used to predict severity — increasing age, high BMI, biliary aetiology, elevated CRP, left-sided pleural effusion are all associated with a poorer prognosis.

However scoring systems which amalgamate various risk factors are much more reliable and there are various acute pancreatitis specific systems — Ranson's score, Imrie's score (Glasgow score) and the Balthazar CT grading system.

f) The complications of acute pancreatitis can be classified as intra-abdominal and systemic. The systemic complications are the failure of various organ systems — ARDS, renal failure, cardiovascular failure and systemic sepsis which usually secondary to intra-abdominal sepsis. The intra-abdominal complications are acute peri-pancreatic fluid collections, pancreatic necrosis, infection within the pancreatic necrosis, development of pseudocysts and vascular complications like formation of pseudoaneurysms mainly of the gastro-duodenal and splenic arteries and portal/splenic vein thrombosis.

Case 3

A 68-year-old retired factory worker has been referred to the hospital with a three-week history of progressively deepening yellow colouration of eyes, dark urine and pale stools. He denies any pain. On examination he is icteric and a smooth mass is felt in the right upper abdomen.

a) What is the most likely diagnosis?
b) What investigations will be of use in confirming this?
c) What is the pathophysiological basis for his symptoms?
d) What are you able to feel on abdominal examination? State the relevant "law".
e) What are the treatment options?

Answers

a) The most likely diagnosis is a malignancy of the head of the pancreas, the most common variety of which is a ductal adeno-carcinoma of pancreas. A distal bile duct neoplasm (cholangio-carcinoma) or an ampullary adenocarcinoma could also occur but they are less common.

b) A triple-phase contrast CT scan of the pancreas is usually able to confirm the diagnosis although endoscopic ultrasound may be necessary.

c) This classical history can be summarised as "painless obstructive jaundice". Dark urine results from urinary excretion of conjugated bilirubin. Pale stools indicate the absence of bile-derived pigments. All these can be explained by biliary obstruction, either intra-hepatic cholestasis (mainly due to drugs and due to severe viral hepatitis when the liver swells within its capsule causing compression of intra-hepatic biliary radicals) or extra-hepatic obstruction to bile flow usually due to calculi or tumours.

d) The smooth palpable abdominal mass is most probably the gall bladder. Courvoisier's law states that — if, in the presence of obstructive jaundice, the gall bladder is palpable, then the cause of jaundice is unlikely to be stones. If the jaundice is due to a common duct stone, then it is likely that recurrent episodes of previous inflammation would have caused fibrosis of the gall bladder wall, which would have prevented the gall bladder from distending to a size that is palpable.

e) Surgical resection of the tumour is the best treatment. However many patients present late and are inoperable (80%). The location of the tumour dictates the type of operation. The most common location of pancreatic ductal adenocarcinoma is the head of the pancreas and the usual operation in this situation is a Pylorus Preserving Pancreatico-Duodenectomy (PPPD). These operations are major procedures and in addition to this being a resectable tumour, the patients have to be fit. For ductal adenocarcinoma, the five-year survival following resection is only 10% to 15%. If this tumour in the head of the pancreas is not operable (usually due to it involving the portal/superior mesenteric veins and/ arteries) then a self-expanding metal stent is used to relieve biliary obstruction. If gastric outflow obstruction is present due to duodenal stenosis (due to tumour growth) then biliary stenting can be combined with laparoscopic gastro-jejunostomy or a double bypass (gastric and biliary) can be performed at open operation. In patients who cannot undergo surgery, chemotherapy can be used but treatment is usually palliative.

Case 4

A 32-year-old male with a long history of intermittent binge drinking is referred by his GP when he develops progressive upper abdominal pain which was initially episodic. The pain is now constant and he has lost about two stones in weight over the past month. On examination there is evidence of recent loss of weight. Abdominal examination is unremarkable.

a) What would your working diagnosis be?
b) What other symptoms could be present?
c) What are the specific investigations of use in this patient?
d) What are the causes for this disease condition?
e) How would you treat him?

Answers

a) The combination of chronic excessive alcohol consumption, upper abdominal pain and weight loss are classical of chronic pancreatitis. This is a disorder of the pancreas characterised by irreversible changes in its parenchyma and its ductal system. The abdominal pain is thought to result from chronic inflammation in the retro-peritoneum and also raised pressure in the pancreatic ductal system. There is loss of both exocrine and endocrine function of the gland causing malabsorption and insulin deficiency.

b) Steatorrhea, that is bulky, greasy, offensive stools which float indicate exocrine deficiency. Insulin deficiency can cause weight loss, polyuria and polydipsia. Jaundice can occur due to biliary stricturing.

c) A fasting blood sugar level, Hb1Ac, nutritional markers such as serum albumin, levels of trace minerals, vitamin B12, folic acid and iron levels. A faecal elastase estimation to confirm pancreatic exocrine deficiency. A triple phase contrast CT scan of the pancreas demonstrates the parenchymal changes. An MRCP can be used to image the ductal system of the pancreas. Endoscopic ultrasound scanning is very sensitive in detecting early changes of chronic pancreatitis and is used in screening for pancreatic cancer in high-risk patients (familial pancreatitis).

d) Chronic excessive alcohol consumption is the main cause (70%). It is increasingly recognised that intermittent binge drinking is as harmful as chronic excessive use. Cholelithiasis only rarely causes chronic pancreatitis. Hereditary pancreatitis is well recognised and is associated with early onset and an increased risk of pancreatic cancer (50 times that of the general population). Tropical pancreatitis is a calcifying condition seen in South India.

Case 5

A 60-year-old woman has just returned from a three-week holiday in Turkey. She has been referred to the outpatient clinic with a history of having developed upper abdominal pain whilst in Turkey which lasted four days. This was associated with a yellow tinge to her eyes and she was generally unwell. All these symptoms have resolved and she is now well.

a) What are the possible diagnoses here?
b) What other points will you elicit on history to further refine your diagnosis?
c) List the investigations you would request and their utility?
d) What is the treatment?
e) What are the significant complications you would watch out for?

Answers

a) The clinical picture of transient painful obstructive jaundice indicates temporary biliary obstruction, most commonly due to the passage of a CBD stone across the ampulla. On occasions a small blood clot (following biliary intervention) or a fragment of a neoplasm can produce the same symptoms.
b) History should be able to distinguish between hepatic and obstructive causes of jaundice. Hepatitis can cause similar symptoms (though the jaundice lasts longer), and in a setting of foreign travel this should be borne in mind.
c) A full haematological and biochemical profile including LFTs are basic. A viral hepatitis screen should be performed. An ultrasound

of the gall bladder will detect gall bladder calculi and the size of the bile ducts both within and outside the liver. An MRCP is the next investigation to look for biliary ductal calculi even if the LFTs are minimally abnormal. An endoscopic ultrasound of the CBD can be performed if the probability of the presence of a CBD stone is high (dilated cuts on USS, elevated bilirubin and liver enzymes). The advantage is that along with diagnosis, an ERCP and extraction of ductal calculi can be performed in the same sitting.

d) If CBD stones are present then the options are between ERCP, sphincterotomy and CBD stone extraction followed by laparoscopic cholecystectomy and laparoscopic cholecystectomy, intra-operative cholangiography and laparoscopic CBD stone extraction.

e) A spiking temperature may indicate the development of cholangitis which can be life-threatening. Acute cholangitis needs urgent treatment with intravenous antibiotics and relief of biliary obstruction by ERCP and further procedures as necessary. Acute pancreatitis is another potential complication.

Extended Matching Questions

EMQ 1

a. Liver function tests
b. Ultrasound scan of abdomen
c. Clotting studies
d. Full blood count
e. Hepatitis viral serology
f. MRCP
g. ERCP
h. CT scan of abdomen
i. Liver biopsy
j. Upper GI endoscopy
k. Faecal elastase
l. Serum amylase

Select the investigation of choice from the list above, which will aid in diagnosis of further management for the following descriptions of patients:

1) A young male presented to his GP with a five-day history of fever and non-specific ill health associated with RUQ pain. His GP found abnormal LFTs and organised an USS of the abdomen, which was normal. The patient has now recovered and has been referred to the hospital for further investigation.

2) An elderly female patient is due to undergo an ERCP the following morning. You have been given a message by the doctor previously on-call to "take a blood test". What will you specifically request?

3) A middle-aged female patient has been admitted through the A&E with obstructive jaundice confirmed biochemically. What is your next investigation?

4) A 70-year-old female presented with back pain and extreme weight loss. Her GP organised an USS, which has suggested a mass in the body of the pancreas.

5) A middle-aged patient with an eight-month history of abnormal LFTs but normal USS and normal MRCP.

6) A young male presents with a 12-hour history of upper abdominal pain. The nurse practitioner in the A&E has organised an erect CXR which is normal. Other routine investigations are awaited. What test will you ensure has been requested?

Answers

1) e.

Viral hepatitis is a common cause of this clinical picture. It would of course be usual that the LFTs would be repeated in the outpatient setting to confirm they had returned to normal.

2) c.

Identification and correction of clotting abnormalities is essential before any invasive procedure.

3) b.

An USS is the first investigation in a patient with jaundice.

4) h.

A CT scan with pancreatic protocol will stage this lesion in the pancreas accurately and will direct further investigation.

5) i.

This patient's history is strongly suggestive of chronic hepatitis as evidenced by LFTs being abnormal for more than six months. A liver biopsy will determine the cause of chronic hepatitis.

6) l.

Acute pancreatitis is high on the list as an alternative diagnosis and a serum amylase estimation will help to diagnose it.

EMQ 2

a. Biliary colic
b. Head of pancreas malignancy
c. Chronic pancreatitis
d. Liver abscess
e. Hepatitis
f. Acute pancreatitis
g. Cholangitis
h. Oesophagitis
i. Mallory-Weiss syndrome

Select the most appropriate diagnosis from the list above for the individual description of patients below:

1) A 70-year-old male is referred with a six-week history of feeling unwell and a week's duration of yellow colouration of the eyes associated with pale stools and dark urine.

2) A 40-year-old publican presents with steatorrhea associated with progressive loss of weight.

3) A middle-aged female reports intermittent episodes of right upper abdominal pain radiating through to the back. Examination is unremarkable.

4) A 55-year-old accountant who works for a financial institution has returned from a six-month period of work in the Africa. He has been suffering intermittent fever associated with chills for the past few weeks. Persistent dull upper abdominal pain has prompted him to seek medical opinion. He is febrile with a tender fullness in the RUQ.

5) A university student has self-presented to the A&E with a 12-hour history of severe epigastric pain radiating to the back associated with numerous episodes of vomiting. He is afebrile but significantly dehydrated and demonstrates tenderness in the epigastrium.

6) A 60-year-old woman who is known to have a benign biliary stricture with a plastic stent in the common bile duct presents with a spiking temperature. On examination she is icteric and has a pulse of 100 beats per minute with a blood pressure of 100/60.

Answers

1) b.
Painless obstructive jaundice usually signifies a malignancy in the region of the head of the pancreas.

2) c.
Chronic pancreatitis can cause both exocrine and endocrine deficiency of the pancreas. The former is manifested by diabetes mellitus and the latter by steatorrhea. Weight loss can be a symptom of both.

3) a.
Cholelithiasis typically causes colicky RUQ pain which radiates posteriorly to the angle of the scapula.

4) d.

A liver abscess is likely. If the abscess is pyogenic, then a search for the cause of the abscess will be needed. Percutaneous drainage and appropriate antibiotics is the initial management.

5) f.

The differential diagnoses here include acute gastritis and a perforated peptic ulcer.

6) g.

Any foreign body in the biliary system predisposes to infection. She will need replacement of the biliary stent.

EMQ 3

a. Laparoscopic cholecystectomy
b. Percutaneous transhepatic cholangiography and biliary drainage (PTC and PTBD)
c. Endoscopic retrograde cholangio-pancreatography (ERCP)
d. Pancreatoduodenectomy (Whipple operation)
e. Insertion of metal biliary stent
f. Palliative treatment
g. Frey's procedure
h. Investigate for other causes of symptoms

With regard to the following patients, select the appropriate treatment from the list above:

1) A localised head of pancreas mass with radiological and cytological features of malignancy.
2) An inoperable mass in the body of the pancreas.
3) A large mass in the head of the pancreas with metastases to the liver causing biliary obstruction.
4) Documented common bile duct stones in a patient who has undergone laparoscopic cholecystectomy 12 years ago.
5) A young woman with lower abdominal pain whose ultrasound scan demonstrates gall bladder stones.

Answers

1) d.
Surgery is the best treatment option, as it affords the best chance of long-term survival. Chemotherapy is mainly used in the palliative setting. However recent trials have demonstrated its usefulness in an adjuvant setting in patients who have undergone a complete resection of the tumour.

2) f.
Pain is a significant symptom in advanced pancreatic malignancies and its relief demands opiates and on occasion procedures such as coeliac plexus block or splanchnicectomy.

3) e.
This patient will invariably have biliary obstruction which is best palliated by a metal stent

4) c.
Laparoscopic bile duct exploration is another option if ERCP fails.

5) h.
Around 15%–20% of the population have asymptomatic gall stones and only one in ten of these will develop symptoms over the five years following the detection of gall bladder stones. Lower abdominal pain is not a manifestation of biliary tract stones.

EMQ 4

a. Progressive weight loss
b. Worsening back pain
c. Rapid worsening of liver function tests
d. Unrelenting RUQ pain in a patient with known gall bladder stones
e. Itching
f. Jaundice associated with fever, chills and rigours in a patient awaiting laparoscopic cholecystectomy
g. Loss of appetite
h. Worsening jaundice
i. Oedema
j. Spiking temperature

Suggest the most relevant symptom from the above list for the following diagnosis:

1) Onset of diabetes in a patient with chronic pancreatitis.
2) Development of hepatocellular carcinoma in a patient with cirrhosis.
3) Development of pancreatic necrosis in a patient being treated for acute pancreatitis.
4) Onset of acute cholecystitis.
5) Onset of cholangitis.
6) Malignant change in chronic pancreatitis.

Answers

1) a.
Progressive weight loss in spite of adequate supplementation of pancreatic exocrine enzymes indicates onset of diabetes. The other cause is development of malignant change in the pancreas.

2) c.
This may be difficult to detect and specialised imaging may be needed — MR/lipoidol CT/contrast enhanced USS.

3) j.
A contrast CT is indicated. Radiological, endoscopic or surgical treatment may be needed.

4) d.
Treatment is conservative either followed by delayed surgery or immediate laparoscopic cholecystectomy.

5) f.
The triad of jaundice, abdominal pain and fever is pathognomonic of cholangitis and aggressive antibiotic treatment along with prompt treatment of the cause is indicated.

6) b.
Back pain is characteristic alongside progressive weight loss. The change to neoplasia from inflammation is difficult to prove and the disease is usually inoperable in these patients.

EMQ 5

a. Insulinoma
b. Hyperlipidaemia
c. Pancreas divisum
d. Adenoma of liver
e. Metastatic carcinoid tumour
f. Haemangioma of liver
g. Cirrhosis
h. Hilar cholangiocarcinoma
i. Multiple endocrine neoplasia-1 (MEN1)

Select the most appropriate diagnosis from the list above for the following clinical presentations:

1) A middle-aged male presents with recurrent episodes of altered behaviour for which he has been laid off from his job as a clerk in a government office. He has high serum C-peptide levels.
2) Dilated intra-hepatic ducts with non-visualisation of the extrahepatic biliary tree on ultrasound scan in a jaundiced 50-year-old previously fit female.
3) Recurrent episodes of acute pancreatitis in a 40-year-old who does not drink alcohol and has no gall stones but has a strong family history of early onset cardiovascular disease.
4) Recurrent sudden episodes of flushing and sensation of warmth all over the body in a patient who has undergone a right hemicolectomy many years ago.
5) A liver mass picked up on ultrasound scanning for lower abdominal pain in a young woman. She has been on the oral contraceptive pill for the past eight years.

Answers

> **1) a.**
> Whipple's triad was described by Allen O. Whipple in the 1930s in order to identify which patients would benefit from surgery for an insulinoma. The three conditions that needed to be met were:
>
> - Symptoms and signs of hypoglycaemia, i.e. confusion, personality changes, tachycardia, seizure, stupor, coma, with or without focal neurologic findings.
> - Blood sugar levels below 50 mg per 100 ml, measured at the time of the symptoms.
> - Recovery from an attack following the administration of glucose.

2) i.

Malignancy of the biliary epithelium is most common in the hilum of the liver. Treatment involves relief of jaundice followed by surgical resection which is usually extremely complex.

3) b.

Biochemical causes of recurrent pancreatitis should always be sought and treated.

4) e.

The primary was probably located in the segment of bowel excised many years ago, but the possibility of a synchronous primary should be investigated.

5) d.

Patient should discontinue hormonal methods of contraception. Adenomas have the potential for malignant change and are prone to bleed spontaneously and therefore need careful surveillance or surgical resection.

Chapter 3   Oesophagus, Stomach and Duodenum

Christopher Streets and Mike Griffin

Multiple Choice Questions

[*Each single best answer (SBA) question comprises a stem and a number of answers. You are asked to decide which single item represents the best answer to the question.*]

1. **One of the following statements is incorrect in relation to "dysphagia"**

   a) Relates to pain on swallowing
   b) Is an "alarm" symptom
   c) Can be due to neurological disorders
   d) May be associated with pulmonary disease
   e) Can be initially investigated with an upper gastrointestinal endoscopy

[Best Answer = a]

Explanation

> Dysphagia is defined as difficulty in swallowing, whilst pain on swallowing is termed odynophagia. Causes can be subdivided into intraluminal (foreign body), mural (carcinoma, benign stricture, scleroderma), extramural (goitre, mediastinal lymph nodes, cardiomegaly) or, least frequently, neurological (stroke) conditions. Dysphagia is considered to be an "alarm" symptom since it may indicate the presence of carcinoma of the oesophagus. If dysphagia results in an inability to swallow liquids or saliva, the patient may aspirate fluid into their respiratory tract. The initial investigation is that of an upper gastrointestinal endoscopy followed by a barium swallow if it is normal.

2. **Achalasia**

   a) Is caused by *Trypanosoma cruzi*
   b) The initial investigation of chioce is a barium swallow
   c) Is a risk factor for adenocarcinoma of the oesophagus

d) May be successfully treated with diet and drugs
e) Perforation of the oesophagus is a risk of surgery

[Best Answer = e]

Explanation

Achalasia of the cardia results from disintegration or absence of Auerbach's myenteric plexus but the cause is not known. A similar pathophysiology exists in Chagas disease which is caused by infection with *Trypanosoma cruzi*. A barium swallow will detect changes in established achalasia — gross distension and tortuosity of the oesophagus as well as a tapering constriction at the lower end (bird's beak). However, the earliest changes are found using oesophageal manometry — lack of peristalsis, high resting pressure and incomplete relaxation of the lower oesophageal sphincter. The condition is a risk factor for squamous cell carcinoma of the oesophagus. Dietary modification and drugs have no role to play in the management of the condition which is treated by either balloon dilatation or surgery (Heller's myotomy). Oesophageal perforation is a risk of both these procedures.

3. Pharyngeal pouch

a) Is a true diverticulum
b) Is a traction diverticulum
c) May present with halitosis
d) Is best diagnosed with upper gastrointestinal endoscopy
e) Usually requires open surgery

[Best Answer = c]

Explanation

A pharyngeal pouch or Zenker's diverticulum is a false pulsion diverticulum occurring through Killian's dehiscence between the inferior constrictor and cricopharyngeus. Collection and stasis of recently swallowed food within the pouch can result in halitosis. It may also present as a mass in the left side of the neck. A barium swallow is the safest way to diagnose the condition since an endoscopy can result in perforation. A linear stapler inserted endoscopically can be used to treat the pouch.

4. **Which of the following statements relating to oesophageal cancer is incorrect?**

   a) Is usually diagnosed at an early stage
   b) Risk factors include smoking and alcohol
   c) Treatment may include radiotherapy or chemotherapy
   d) Is predominantly adenocarcinoma in the United Kingdom
   e) Dysphagia and weight loss are poor prognostic signs

[Best Answer = a]

Explanation

Unfortunately it often presents late. The two major histological types of oesophageal cancer are squamous cell carcinoma (SCC) and adenocarcinoma (AC). Whilst worldwide SCC is the more common (China, Iran, South Africa), AC is more prevalent in the West and is increasing in incidence. Risk factors include alcohol, tobacco, achalasia, scleroderma, vitamin A and C deficiencies, dietary toxins for SCC, and gastro-oesophageal reflux disease (GORD), Barrett's oesophagus for AC. Oesophageal cancer often only presents with symptoms (progressive dysphagia, regurgitation, cough, hoarseness, pain, weight loss, and fatigue) when locally advanced. Depending upon the stage of the disease surgery, chemotherapy and radiotherapy are all possible treatment modalities.

5. **Hiatus hernia**

   a) Is an uncommon finding
   b) Is caused by stomach herniating through the membranous part of the diaphragm
   c) The rolling type is more commonly associated with reflux
   d) The rolling or paraoesophageal type is best managed conservatively
   e) Often co-exists with diverticular disease and gall stones

[Best Answer = e]

Explanation

> Hiatus hernia is common, especially in women, and with advancing years. It results from herniation of the stomach through the oesophageal hiatus of the diaphragm due to laxity of the crura. There are two main types — sliding (80%) and rolling (20%). The sliding type is more likely to be related to symptoms of gastro-oesophageal reflux (i.e. heartburn and regurgitation), while the rolling type may cause pain due to incarceration, ischaemia and gangrene. A sliding hiatus hernia usually can be treated conservatively, but a rolling type needs surgical correction to prevent potentially life-threatening complications. Saint's triad includes the presence of gallstones, diverticular disease and hiatus hernia in the same patient.

6. Oesophageal varices

a) May occur after portal vein thrombosis
b) Commonly bleed after vomiting and retching
c) Are the most common cause of upper gastrointestinal haemorrhage in cirrhotic patients
d) Should be treated on diagnosis
e) Often require surgical procedures to prevent major bleeding

[Best Answer = a]

Explanation

> Oesophageal varices result from portal venous hypertension, causes of which include cirrhosis of the liver due to alcohol abuse, portal vein thrombosis, schistosomiasis and hepatic vein thrombosis (Budd-Chiari syndrome). Large submucosal veins appear at the lower end of the oesophagus which can bleed after minimal trauma from passing food boluses. Even in cirrhotic patients the most common cause of upper gastrointestinal haemorrhage is from peptic ulceration. Small varices do not need treatment but larger ones may require a B-blocker and banding to prevent bleeding. Treatment for haemorrhage includes resuscitation, tamponade with a Minnesota or Sengstaken tube, or

transjugular intrahepatic portosystemic shunting (TIPS). Surgery is rarely required. Child's criteria considers encephalopathy, ascites, bilirubin, albumin and prothrombin ratio in the patient with cirrhosis.

7. Regarding peptic ulceration

a) *Helicobacter pylori* is a Gram-positive bacillus
b) The duodenum is more commonly affected than the stomach
c) Zollinger-Ellison syndrome is associated with gastric hyposecretion
d) H2 receptor antagonists will heal 50% of duodenal ulcers within eight weeks
e) Gastric ulcers are rarely malignant

[Best Answer = b]

Explanation

Helicobacter pylori is a flagellated Gram-negative bacillus and is thought to be associated with 90% of duodenal ulcers and 80% of gastric ulcers. Other risk factors include cigarette smoking, alcohol, NSAIDs and stress. Duodenal ulcers occur more commonly than gastric ulcers. A gastric cancer may initially present as a gastric ulcer. Zollinger-Ellison syndrome results from a rare gastrin-secreting tumour that produces severe peptic ulceration extending into and even beyond the second part of the duodenum. Medical treatment of peptic ulceration includes H2 receptor antagonists (cimetidine, ranitidine, famotidine), proton pump inhibitors (omeprazole, lansoprazole, pantoprazole, rabeprazole, esomeprazole) and *Helicobacter pylori* eradication. H2 receptor antagonists will heal 90% of duodenal ulcers within eight weeks and triple therapy can eradicate *Helicobacter pylori* in 80% of patients within one week. Surgery is rarely indicated.

8. Gastric cancer

a) Is increasing in incidence
b) Is not associated with *Helicobacter pylori* infection
c) Is best treated by radiotherapy or chemotherapy

d) May present with a Krukenberg tumour
e) Fundal lesions are more common than antral lesions

[Best Answer = d]

Explanation

> The incidence of gastric cancer is 23 per 100,000 per year with a peak during the fifth and sixth decades. Risk factors include *Helicobacter pylori* infection, blood group A, high salt and nitrate intake, and deficiency of vitamins A, C and E. Treatment usually consists of neoadjuvant chemotherapy followed by surgery and then a course of adjuvant chemotherapy. Transcoelomic spread to the ovaries results in a Krukenberg tumour. Antral lesions are more common than fundal lesions, leading to symptoms of gastric outlet obstruction (early satiety and vomiting).

9. Intrinsic factor

a) Is a polysaccharide
b) Is produced by the parietal cells in the pancreas
c) Acts in the terminal ileum
d) Is important in the absorption of folic acid
e) Deficiency can be treated with oral vitamin B12

[Best Answer = c]

Explanation

> Intrinsic factor is a glycoprotein secreted by the parietal cells present in the gastric body mucosa. It is necessary for the absorption of vitamin B12 (cyanocobalamin). Vitamin B12 binds to intrinsic factor in the intestinal lumen and allows its transfer across the terminal ileum into the blood stream. Any state in which the parietal cells are absent (e.g. gastrectomy) or not functioning properly (e.g. pernicious anaemia) can result in reduced secretion of intrinsic factor and thus vitamin B12 deficiency. Vitamin B12 must be administered intramuscularly in such patients.

10. One of the following statements is incorrect in relation to Coeliac disease

a) It results from dietary lactose intolerance
b) It is associated with raised serum anti-endomysial and anti-gliadin antibodies
c) Small bowel histology usually shows villous hypertrophy
d) Increases the risk of small bowel lymphoma
e) Can be effectively treated with a gluten-free diet

[Best Answer = a]

Explanation

Coeliac disease is a malabsorption syndrome and results from a congenital absence of gluten hydrolase in the small bowel mucosal cells. There is intolerance to gluten, a protein present in wheat, rye, barley and oats, resulting in the build-up of the metabolite gliadin in the mucosal cells. Small bowel mucosal villous atrophy ensues which can be seen in biopsies taken at endoscopy. Coeliac disease increases the risk of small bowel lymphoma but can be treated by adherence to a gluten-free diet.

11. Small bowel obstruction

a) In the United Kingdom, is most often due to an obstructed hernia
b) Causes absent bowel sounds, colicky abdominal pain and diarrhoea
c) Abdominal distension is seen in all patients
d) Often requires aggressive intravenous fluid resuscitation
e) All cases can be managed conservatively for the initial 24 hours

[Best Answer = d]

Explanation

The incidence of small bowel obstruction increases with the frequency of abdominal surgery. Therefore in the developed world (e.g. Europe, North America) the most common cause is adhesions from previous abdominal surgery, in underdeveloped countries it is obstructed hernia. Colicky abdominal pain is the cardinal symptom with vomiting being present in all but very distal small bowel obstruction associated with distension and absolute constipation. The more proximal the lesion, the earlier vomiting occurs. Abdominal distension may be absent in a proximal obstruction. The vomiting and intestinal ileus can result in huge fluid shifts and electrolyte disturbances which will require many litres of intravenous fluid to correct. Whilst many cases of adhesional obstruction will settle with conservative management (i.e. nasogastric tube, intravenous fluids), those that develop pain, pyrexia, tachycardia and signs of peritonism will need surgery.

12. Meckel's diverticulum

a) Occurs in 10% of the population
b) Will be found in the mesenteric border of the small intestine
c) Consists of mucosa without a muscle coat
d) A fibrous band between its apex and the liver can result in intestinal obstruction
e) Heterotopic gastric mucosa can ulcerate and cause a brisk gastrointestinal bleed

[Best Answer = e]

Explanation

A Meckel's diverticulum is a remnant of the intestinal end of the vitello-intestinal duct. It is present in about 2% of the population, is two inches long and arises from the anti-mesenteric border of the ileum, two feet proximal to the ileo-caecal valve. It is a true diverticulum containing all layers of the bowel. In 10% of cases a fibrous band, the remainder of the vitello-intestinal duct, connects it to the umbilicus and may be a cause of intestinal obstruction. Fifty per cent of symptomatic Meckel's diverticula contain heterotopic tissue. If this is parietal cell gastric mucosa, peptic ulceration and associated complications can occur.

13. Carcinoid tumour

a) Most commonly affect the colon
b) Symptoms of carcinoid syndrome usually occur before metastases have arisen
c) Carcinoid syndrome occurs once lung metastases have occurred
d) Urinary 5-HIAA is elevated in patients with carcinoid syndrome
e) Surgery is deemed inappropriate once the tumour has metastasised

[Best Answer = d]

Explanation

The appendix is the most common site of gastrointestinal carcinoid formation followed by the small bowel. Whilst one third of the tumours will have metastasised at presentation, only 10% of patients present with carcinoid syndrome. Usually the secretory products (e.g. 5-hydroxytryptamine, prostaglandins, kinins) of the tumour are inactivated by the liver, but liver metastases are able to secrete directly into the systemic circulation causing carcinoid syndrome. The symptoms consist of periodic facial flushing, diarrhoea, and asthmatic attacks whilst the majority of patients with the syndromes have elevated levels of 5-hydroxyindoleacetic acid (5-HIAA). Treatment of carcinoid tumours involves radical excision of all the accessible tumour. Partial hepatic lobectomy can be employed if metastases are localised.

14. Initial treatment of an enterocutaneous fistula includes

a) Enteral nutrition
b) Neostigmine
c) Laparoscopic resection
d) Skin grafting
e) Octreotide

[Best Answer = e]

Explanation

Although 90% of enterocutaneous fistulae are a complication of surgery, some may occur spontaneously (e.g. Crohn's disease). Fistulae are classified according to the amount of fluid lost through them — "high output" or "low output". Treatment includes maintaining fluid and electrolyte balance, control of sepsis (antibiotics) and ensuring adequate drainage, nutritional support (total parenteral nutrition), exclusion of distal obstruction (may require surgery), and skin care. The volume of gastrointestinal secretions can be reduced using octreotide, a somatostatin analogue.

15. Gallstone ileus

a) Results from a gallstone impacting at the ileo-caecal junction
b) Is a rare cause of large bowel obstruction
c) Air in the biliary tree can sometimes be seen on plain radiographs
d) Is treated by cholecystectomy
e) At surgery the gallstone is simply milked into the caecum

[Best Answer = c]

Explanation

Gallstone ileus is a rare cause of small bowel obstruction arising from the passage of a gallstone through a cholecystoduodenal fistula. The stone classically impacts at the narrowest part of the small bowel some two feet proximal to the ileo-caecal junction. This is the point at which the vitello-intestinal duct would have joined the ileum. Air can pass from the duodenum through the fistula into the biliary tree (aerobilia) and may be evident on plain chest and abdominal radiographs. At surgery an enterotomy is made proximal to the point of impaction and the gallstone removed through it. The cholecystoduodenal fistula can usually be left alone.

Case Studies

Case 1

A 64-year-old man presents with a three-month history of difficulty swallowing. Initially he had problems with meat and bread however more recently he has experienced difficulty with liquids. He has lost 10 kg in weight over that period.

a) What are the causes of dysphagia?
b) What are the symptoms and signs of oesophageal cancer?
c) How should this patient be investigated?
d) What is the surgical management of oesophageal cancer?
e) What is the role of chemotherapy and radiotherapy in the treatment of oesophageal cancer?
f) What are the complications of oesophagectomy?

Answers

a) Obstructive causes of dysphagia may be caused by luminal or extraluminal causes. Luminal — oesophagitis, webs and benign or malignant strictures. Extraluminal — Zenkers diverticulum, mediastinal masses, enlarged thyroid, vertebral osteophytes, aberrant right subclavian artery, left atrial hypertrophy, aortic aneurysm or right sided aorta. Oesophageal motility may cause dysphagia — muscle weakness, achalasia, diffuse oesophageal spasm and systemic sclerosis.

b) Early oesophageal cancer is often asymptomatic with no physical signs. More advanced cancer can result in progressive dysphagia initially to solids, then to liquids, regurgitation, aspiration, hoarseness, pain, weight loss and fatigue. Signs of metastatic disease include supraclavicular lymphadenopathy, hepatomegaly, recurrent laryngeal nerve palsy and bronchopulmonary complications.

c) An urgent upper gastrointestinal endoscopy is mandatory. This enables localisation of the tumour position and biopsies for histological confirmation. Once the diagnosis of oesophageal carcinoma (adeno or squamous cell) has been made the patient's disease needs to be staged. A CT scan of the chest, abdomen and pelvis will determine the presence of distant metastases (M stage) and lymph nodes (N stage). An endoscopic ultrasound scan will determine the stage of the tumour (T stage) and local lymph nodes (N stage). Bronchoscopy may also be considered if airway involvement is suspected. The general fitness of the patients to be assessed prior to definitive treatment and haematological, biochemical, cardiac and pulmonary investigations will be used.

d) Approximately 30% of patients are suitable for oesophageactomy. The three approaches are an Ivor Lewis oesophagectomy (laparotomy and right thoracotomy) for a mid or low tumour, a transthoracic or thoracoabdominal approach (left thoracotomy) for a low tumour, and a transhiatal oesophagectomy (laparotomy and left cervical incision) for an upper tumour. A radical lymphadenectomy is also performed.

e) Chemotherapy may be given palliatively or in a neoadjuvant setting with good effect. Squamous cell carcinomas are more radiosensitive than adenocarcinomas and so chemoradiotherapy may be used as primary treatment in the former group. Radiotherapy may be used palliatively.

f) The operative mortality from oesophagectomy is less than 5% in tertiary centres of excellence, with a morbidity of 40%. Complications include anastomotic leak and stricture, wound and chest infection, pleural effusion, chylothorax, intra-abdominal abscess, haemorrhage, splenic injury, recurrent laryngeal nerve palsy, necrosis of the gastric conduit and delayed gastric emptying.

Case 2

A 40-year-old man has a four-year history of heartburn. It is particularly bad when lying down at night and is made worse by bending over. Occasionally he is awoken at night by coughing and choking. Over-the-counter antacids provide some relief. His general practitioner has diagnosed him as having gastro-oesophageal reflux disease (GORD).

a) What are the clinical features of GORD?
b) What is the pathophysiology of GORD?
c) What are the complications of GORD?
d) What is the initial investigation of choice?
e) How can GORD be treated?
f) What are the possible complications of surgery?

Answers

a) The typical symptoms of GORD are heartburn, regurgitation and dysphagia. Atypical symptoms include retrosternal chest pain, hoarseness, hiccups, ear pain, loss of dental enamel, night sweats, chronic wheeze or cough, globus sensation, hypersalivation and halitosis.

b) A small degree of gastro-oesophageal reflux is physiological but once the presence of gastric juice results in symptoms or complications (e.g. oesophagitis, stricture, Barrett's metaplasia) it is termed pathological. Failure of oesophageal, gastric and duodenal protective mechanisms are responsible for GORD; oesophageal — loss of the high pressure zone of the lower oesophageal sphincter, reduced oesophageal peristalsis, and decreased salivary and oesophageal mucosal bicarbonate production; gastric — gastric distension, increased intra-abdominal pressure; duodenal — alkaline reflux.

c) Prolonged exposure of the oesophageal mucosa to gastric juice may result in inflammation, erosions, ulceration and stricture. Metaplasia of the lower oesophagus may occur with replacement of the normal squamous epithelium by columnar intestinal epithelium (Barrett's oesophagus). This condition is premalignant and can lead to dysplasia and cancer.

d) An upper gastrointestinal endoscopy is the initial test to assess the extent and severity of the disease. The endoscopy also allows biopsies to be taken if necessary.

e) Initial lifestyle changes include weight loss, cessation of smoking, avoiding foodstuffs that precipitate symptoms, not eating a large meal late at night and elevating the head of the bed. Medical treatment involves antacids or alginates, H2 receptor antagonists (cimetidine, ranitidine, nizatidine and famotidine), proton pump inhibitors (omeprazole, lansoprazole, pantoprazole, rabeprazole and esomeprazole) and prokinetic agents (metoclromide, domperidone and erythromycin). Surgery includes open or laparoscopic fundoplication. After closure of the hiatal defect the mobilised fundus is wrapped to a various extend around the lower oesophagus either posteriorly or anteriorly.

Case 3

A 32-year-old female attends the A&E department vomiting bright red blood and feeling faint. She was commenced on a course of diclofenac for back pain three weeks ago and has experienced indigestion ever since. She smokes 20 cigarettes a day and drinks occasionally.

a) How should this patient initially be managed?
b) What are the causes of upper gastrointestinal haemorrhage?
c) What are the risk factors for peptic ulcer disease?
d) What are the complications of peptic ulcer disease?
e) What is meant by "triple-therapy"?
f) What are the alternatives to medical management of peptic ulcer disease?

Answers

a) This patient is in shock from an upper gastrointestinal haemorrhage and requires resuscitation. Oxygen needs to be administered via a face mask with a reservoir bag at 15 litres per minute, and two wide bore intravenous cannulae inserted for the immediate infusion of two litres of normal saline. Blood must be sent for urgent cross-matching of six units of red blood cells as well as full blood count, coagulation, and urea and electrolytes. A urinary catheter and nasogastric tube need to be inserted. Arrangements must be made for an emergency upper gastrointestinal endoscopy.

b) Most upper gastrointestinal haemorrhages are from gastric or duodenal ulcers. Other causes are oesophagitis, oesophageal or gastric varices, Mallory-Weiss tear, acute erosive gastritis, gastric angiodysplasia, Dieulafoy's malformation, duodenitis and tumours.

c) There is a very strong association between the presence of *Helicobacter pylori* and peptic ulceration — 95% of duodenal and 70%–80% of gastric ulcers. Other risk factors include non-steroidal anti-inflammatory drugs, steroids, cigarette smoking, alcohol, blood group O and Zollinger-Ellison syndrome. Curling's ulcers are associated with major body surface burns. Cushing's ulcers are associated with head injuries.

d) The main complications of upper gastrointestinal ulcers are haemorrhage (haematemesis, melaena, iron deficiency anaemia), perforation, and obstruction (pyloric stenosis).

e) The long-term healing of gastric or duodenal ulcers can be rapidly achieved by eradicating *Helicobacter pylori*, the causative factor in many cases. A "triple-therapy" regimen is a combination of a proton pump inhibitor (e.g. lansoprazole) and two antibiotics (e.g. amoxicillin and clarithromycin) administered for one week. It is efficacious in 80%–90% of cases.

f) With the advent of the proton pump inhibitors elective surgery for peptic ulcer disease is rarely indicated. Zollinger-Ellison syndrome must be excluded in patients with duodenal ulcers refractory to medical treatment. Selective vagotomy and antrectomy, or subtotal gastrectomy may be employed with refractory duodenal ulcers. Refractory gastric ulcers are even rarer, but when they do occur may be treated with either excision of the ulcer accompanied by a highly selective vagotomy or a subtotal gastrectomy.

Case 4

A 73-year-old woman presents with anorexia, early satiety and significant weight loss. The symptoms have gradually worsened over the previous three months. She is otherwise fit and well but has been found to have iron deficiency anaemia.

a) What is the differential diagnosis for this lady?
b) What are the risk factors for gastric cancer?
c) How should this patient be evaluated?
d) What eponymous signs are related to the metastatic spread of gastric cancer?
e) What are the surgical options for managing the patient?
f) What are the complications of surgery?

Answers

a) Considering this woman's age and symptoms an upper gastrointestinal tract neoplasm, in particular gastric cancer, needs to be excluded. Peptic ulcer disease can also present with similar symptoms.

b) Risk factors for gastric cancer include — chronic atrophic gastritis and intestinal metaplasia; pernicious anaemia; gastric remnant (a cancer arising in the remaining stomach after a previous gastric resection); adenomatous gastric polyps; gastric ulcers (especially non-healing ones); *Helicobacter pylori* infection.

c) Upper gastrointestinal endoscopy enables a histological diagnosis to be made. A CT scan of the chest, abdomen and pelvis will identify any nodal (N stage) and haematogenous metastatic spread typically to the liver or the lungs (M stage). An endoscopic ultrasound scan will assess the depth of gastric wall invasion (T stage) and local lymph node involvement (N stage). A staging laparoscopy will also be required to detect peritoneal spread of the cancer.

d) Virchow's node or Troisier's sign — a palpable lymph node in the left supraclavicular fossa. Irish's node — a palpable node in the left axilla. Sister Mary Joseph's node — a metastatic nodule in the umbilicus. Krukenberg's tumour — ovarian metastases. Blumer's shelf — pelvic peritoneal metastases that are palpable during a rectal or pelvic examination.

e) A surgical technique aimed at curing gastric cancer must consider the amount of stomach removed to obtain local clearance, the degree of nodal dissection and the method of reconstruction. Proximal cancers are best managed with a radical total gastrectomy — *en-bloc* removal of the omentum, stomach, first part of duodenum, and surrounding lymph nodes. A distal cancer is managed by a radical subtotal gastrectomy — *en-bloc* resection of the omentum, 80% of the stomach, first part of the duodenum and surrounding lymph nodes. In the past Billroth I (duodenal stump anastomosed to remainder of the stomach) or Billroth II (duodenal stump oversewn and gastric remnant anastomosed to proximal jejunum) reconstructions have been used, but a Roux-en-Y technique is now preferred.

f) Operative mortality should be less than 8% for a total gastrectomy and 5% for a subtotal gastrectomy. Early complications include bleeding, infection and anastomotic leak. Later complications include vitamin B_{12} deficiency, anaemia, metabolic bone disease, blind loop syndrome, chronic diarrhoea, and early and late dumping syndromes.

Case 5

A 55-year-old man presents with a four-day history of colicky abdominal pain and vomiting. Over the last two days he has not opened his bowels and he has not passed flatus for 24 hours. In the past he underwent an appendicectomy for perforated appendicitis.

a) What is the probable diagnosis?
b) What are the common causes of small bowel obstruction?
c) What are the physical findings in small bowel obstruction?
d) What abnormalities might be found on initial investigations?
e) What is the initial treatment of a patient with small bowel obstruction?
f) What are the indications for surgery?

Answers

a) This patient has small bowel obstruction until proven otherwise. Other diagnoses include ileus, large bowel obstruction, volvulus, gastroenteritis, pancreatitis and mesenteric ischaemia.

b) Post-operative adhesions account for up to two-thirds of small bowel obstruction, with incarcerated hernia and neoplasm being the next most common causes. Less common causes include diverticulitis, gallstone ileus and inflammatory bowel disease.

c) The most common findings in the patient with small bowel obstruction relate to dehydration — tachycardia, dry mucous membranes and reduced skin turgor. Usually abdominal examination is unremarkable with moderate discomfort. Scars and hernial orifices need to be examined carefully.

d) Vomiting and sequestration of fluid within the loops of small bowel can result in dehydration. Haematocrit and urea may be raised. There may be a hypochloraemic hypokalaemic metabolic acidosis due to vomiting. A plain abdominal radiograph may show multiple loops of distended small bowel with absence of air in the colon. If the film is taken in the upright position air-fluid levels will be seen in these loops of small bowel. An erect chest radiograph should be examined for the presence of free gas under the diaphragm in the case of perforation.

e) A nasogastric tube is inserted to decompress the stomach. Aggressive intravenous fluid therapy is required to address the dehydration. To monitor the effect a urinary catheter is inserted aiming for a urine output of 0.5 ml per kg per hour. A frail elderly patient with cardiac co-morbidities may require central venous pressure monitoring. The response to intravenous fluid therapy and the general condition of the patient needs to be continually re-assessed.

f) Surgery is required for bowel strangulation, closed-loop obstruction and ischaemic bowel. Increasing abdominal tenderness, fever, raised white blood cell count, acidosis, peritoneal irritation and shock are all signs of bowel necrosis. However, even without these worrying clinical signs unresolving small bowel obstruction usually necessitates an operation.

Extended Matching Questions

EMQ 1

a. Stroke
b. Scleroderma
c. Candidiasis
d. Boerhaave's syndrome
e. Achalasia
f. Oesophageal cancer
g. Gastro-oesophageal reflux disease
h. Gastric cancer
i. Small bowel obstruction
j. Crohn's disease

From the list above choose the most likely diagnosis for the following clinical situations:

1) A 40-year-old lady complaining of intermittent dysphagia to liquids more than solids with Raynaud's phenomenon.
2) A 60-year-old man with vomiting, abdominal distension and a tender non-reducible lump in his right groin.
3) A 70-year-old man with severe indigestion, weight loss, a palpable mass in his epigstrium and palpable left supraclavicular lymphadenopathy.
4) A 55-year-old man who experiences severe chest pain after repeated vomiting and retching.
5) A 35-year-old man presenting with heartburn and regurgitation.

Answers

1) b.
This patient has systemic sclerosis or scleroderma. The signs and symptoms can be remembered by CREST: Calcinosis — calcium deposits in the skin; Raynaud's phenomenon — spasm of the blood vessels in response to cold or stress; Esophageal dysfunction — acid reflux and decreased motility of the oesophagus; Sclerodactyly — thickening and tightening of the skin on the fingers and hands; and Telangiectasia — dilatation of capillaries causing red marks on the surface of the skin. A minimum of two is needed to make the diagnosis.

2) i.

This man has an incarcerated inguinal hernia resulting in small bowel obstruction.

3) h.

An advanced gastric cancer will produce a palpable mass in the upper abdomen. An involved left supraclavicular node is called a Virchow's node which is referred to as Troisier's sign.

4) d.

Repeated vomiting may rupture the lower oesophagus and cause gastric contents to contaminate the mediastinum. Pleural effusions and empyemas may also develop.

5) g.

These are the typical symptoms of gastro-oesophageal reflux disease.

EMQ 2

Options

a. CT scan
b. Angiography
c. Endoscopy
d. Barium swallow
e. Gastric emptying study
f. Meckel's scan
g. Barium meal
h. MRI scan
i. Oesophageal manometry
j. Ambulatory 24-hour pHmetry

Choose an answer from the list above which is the most appropriate initial investigation for the following patients:

1) An 84-year-old female with intermittent dysphagia to solids and a normal endoscopy.
2) A 50-year-old man presenting with light headedness and melaena.
3) A 35-year-old man with repeated episodes of melaena and a normal endoscopy.
4) A 65-year-old man with progressive dysphagia and weight loss.

5) A 40-year-old woman with intermittent progressive dysphagia to liquids in particular. She also experiences regurgitation of undigested food.

Answers

1) d.
The normal endoscopy has ruled out any mucosal cause for the dysphagia such as cancer or oesophagitis. The barium swallow will demonstrate the oesophageal dysmotility resulting in the symptoms (i.e. poor peristalsis, tertiary contractions and "yo-yoing" of the bread bolus. This lady will have the non-specific oesophageal motility disorder called presbyoesophagus.

2) c.
Melaena implies bleeding from the upper gastrointestinal tract and if the patient feels faint a significant quantity of blood has been lost. Peptic ulceration is the most common cause of such bleeding and an urgent endoscopy is the most appropriate investigation. A bleeding gastric or duodenal ulcer can also be treated at endoscopy (e.g. adrenaline injection, diathermy or heater probe).

3) f.
A Meckel's diverticulum may contain heterotopic gastric mucosa which can ulcerate and bleed. The parietal cells present in this mucosa concentrate 99mTc-sodium pertechnetate which can be detected by scintiscanning (i.e. a Meckel's scan).

4) c.
This man has the "alarm" symptoms of dysphagia and weight loss in a person who is older than 55 years of age. He needs an urgent endoscopy to identify an oesophageal cancer. Not only can the position of the tumour be located but a biopsy can be taken to enable histological confirmation.

5) d.
Achalasia, due to absent oesophageal peristalsis and poor relaxation of the lower oesophageal sphincter, may cause intermittent dysphagia, regurgitation and retrosternal chest pain. A barium swallow will demonstrate a distended oesophagus above a smooth distal narrowing (i.e. bird's beak deformity).

EMQ 3

a. Radical total gastrectomy
b. Endoscopic haemostasis
c. *Helicobacter pylori* eradication therapy
d. Roux en-Y anastomosis
e. Heller's myotomy
f. Small bowel resection
g. Nissen fundoplication
h. Under-running of a bleeding duodenal ulcer
i. Pyloric stent and palliative chemotherapy
j. Oesophagectomy

Select the most appropriate treatment for the following patients from the above list:

1) A 79-year-old man with gastric outlet obstruction from an adenocarcinoma and severe COAD. His staging CT has demonstrated liver metastases.
2) A 40-year-old woman with a longstanding history of dyspepsia. At upper gastrointestinal endoscopy moderate duodenitis was seen and a urease test was positive.
3) A proximal gastric adenocarcinoma in a previously fit and well 64-year-old man. Staging investigations have demonstrated no local nodal or distant haematogenous metastases.
4) A 29-year-old man has had several years of heartburn and regurgitation. His symptoms are improved but not completely relieved by a proton pump inhibitor. He does not wish to take tablets for the rest of his life.
5) A 44-year-old woman who has been diagnosed with achalasia.

Answers

1) i.
This patient has incurable gastric cancer and his symptoms would be best palliated by a pyloric stent and chemotherapy. The former can be placed endoscopically.

2) c.
A positive urease test confirms the presence of *Helicobacter pylori* in the stomach, a significant risk factor for peptic ulcer disease. Eradication of the organism will most likely cure the woman's symptoms.

3) a.

This man appears to be fit enough to undergo a gastrectomy for his cancer. Its proximal location requires a total gastrectomy. A radical procedure will involve *en-bloc* removal of the omentum, stomach, first part of duodenum, and surrounding lymph nodes. It is the best hope of cure. If lymph node metastases were detected by the pre-operative staging investigations, neoadjuvant chemotherapy would be considered.

4) g.

Antireflux surgery would be appropriate in this patient. After suitable pre-operative investigations, a Nissen fundoplication (360°) would be appropriate. Most surgeons would perform this procedure laparoscopically.

5) e.

Achalasia is a motor disorder of the oesophagus resulting in aperistalsis of the oesophagus with a hypertensive, incompletely relaxing lower oesophageal sphincter. A Heller's myotomy of the lower oesophageal sphincter aims to relieve the symptom of dysphagia. It can however result in reflux symptoms and so is commonly combined with a partial fundoplication. The procedure is usually carried out laparoscopically.

EMQ 4

a. Anastomotic leak
b. Wound infection
c. Deep vein thrombosis
d. Chyle leak
e. Pneumothorax
f. Pleural effusion
g. Duodenal stump leak
h. Dumping syndrome
i. Vitamin B_{12} deficiency
j. Gas bloat syndrome

Which of the above postoperative complications apply to the following clinical scenarios?

1) The feeling of upper abdominal fullness and inability to belch after a laparoscopic Nissen fundoplication.

2) Two days following an oesophagectomy, milky-coloured fluid starts to appear in the chest drains. Its volume increases as the patients enteral feeding is commenced.

3) Bile-stained fluid appears in the right abdominal drain a few days after a subtotal gastrectomy.

4) Having re-established oral nutrition after a total gastrectomy the patient experiences episodes of dizziness, palpitations, sweating and diarrhoea immediately after eating.

5) Two and a half years after a subtotal gastrectomy a patient presents to their general practitioner with fatique. Clinically they are anaemic and a blood test confirms this. Their MCV is elevated.

Answers

1) j.
Patients post a Nissen fundoplication (360° wrap) are unable to belch swallowed air. This accumulates in the stomach giving a bloated or distended sensation. This is gas bloat syndrome.

2) d.
The thoracic duct may be damaged during mobilisation of the oesophagus. Chyle is white in colour due to its high fat content. Small leaks will settle spontaneously especially if the enteral feed is changed to medium chain triglycerides. Larger leaks will require surgical re-exploration and ligation.

3) g.
It is generally recommended that a drain be positioned adjacent to the duodenal stump to detect this complication. Early leaks are due to technical error, small bowel obstruction or ischaemia. Early re-exploration is required.

4) h.
This is early dumping syndrome. These symptoms are associated with gastric bloating and are related to the osmotic effect of a large carbohydrate load in the small intestine. Symptoms are best managed by small frequent meals consisting of low carbohydrate and high protein content.

EMQ 5

a. Plummer-Vinson syndrome
b. Dysphagia lusoria
c. Myasthenia gravis
d. Rolling hiatus hernia
e. Zenker's diverticulum
f. Sliding hiatus hernia
g. Zollinger-Ellison syndrome
h. Oesophageal varices
i. Boerhaave's syndrome
j. Mallory-Weiss tear

For each of the following conditions select the most appropriate answer above:

1) An intramural cause of dysphagia.
2) A systemic cause of dysphagia.
3) The most common type of hiatus hernia.
4) A cause of widespread peptic ulceration.
5) Presents as mediastinitis after vomiting.

Answers

1) a.
Plummer-Vinson syndrome. This is the development of an oesophageal web in the presence of iron deficiency, most commonly seen in females of middle age or above. Other intramural causes include malignancy and scleroderma. Zenker's diverticulum (pharyngeal pouch) is regarded as an extramural cause of dysphagia.

2) c.
Myasthenia gravis, can affect swallowing as can other systemic disorders such as Parkinson's disease.

3) f.

Sliding hiatus hernia. This constitutes 85% of hiatus hernias with 10% being rolling and 5% mixed.

4) g.

Zollinger-Ellison syndrome. This is the hyper-secretion of gastric acid due to a gastrin-producing tumour (gastrinoma). The classic feature of Zollinger–Ellison syndrome is refractory peptic ulceration, which may involve the whole duodenum and even small bowel.

5) i.

Boerhaave's syndrome. This is spontaneous rupture of the oesophagus occurring after forceful or prolonged vomiting. It results in mediastinitis (infection and inflammation of the mediastinum as a result of food/fluid/microorganisms entering the mediastinum) and is usually fatal if not promptly treated.

Chapter 4   Colon Rectum and Anus

Doug Aitken and Alan Horgan

Multiple Choice Questions

[Each single best answer (SBA) question comprises a stem and a number of answers. You are asked to decide which single item represents the best answer to the question.]

1. Rectal cancer

a)   Is normally an adenocarcinoma
b)   Usually presents with anaemia
c)   Usually arises in hyperplastic polyps
d)   Is rare compared to colon cancer
e)   Synchronous tumours occur in 20% of patients

[Best Answer = a]

Explanation

Rectal cancers are almost always adenocarcinoma; anal cancers, arising below the dentate line are usually squamous. Between 40% and 50% of colorectal cancers arise in the rectum, usually within adenomatous polyps. Anaemia is a more common presentation of right-sided colon cancer, whereas left-sided lesions tend to present with altered bowel habit, rectal bleeding, or obstructive symptoms. About 3% of patients will have synchronous tumours (another primary tumour that presents at the same time); also 3% will develop metachronous (another primary tumour presenting later) cancers.

2. Fissure-in-ano

a)   Is premalignant
b)   Respond rarely to topical glycerol trinitrate (GTN)
c)   Are mainly laterally located
d)   Usually require surgical intervention
e)   Can be treated using botulinum toxin

[Best Answer = e]

Explanation

Most fissures occur in the midline more often posteriorly, and are a common cause of painful defecation. They are not pre-malignant! No treatment may be required, as many fissures will resolve spontaneously; medical therapies should always be tried before surgery. Several topical agents have proved effective in the treatment of fissures, including GTN and calcium channel blockers (e.g. nifedipine). Temporary paralysis of the sphincter muscles with botulinum toxin has also been used successfully.

3. When considering haemorrhoids

a) Prolapse requiring digital reduction characterises grade II disease
b) Rectal bleeding is always present
c) Grade I and II haemorrhoids can be successfully treated without surgery
d) Rubber band ligation is less effective than injection sclerotherapy
e) Iron deficiency anaemia is a common finding

[Best Answer = c]

Explanation

While most patients with haemorrhoids complain of rectal bleeding it is not universally present, other presenting symptoms include pain, or prolapse on defecation. Bleeding sufficient to cause anaemia is uncommon. Grade II haemorrhoids reduce spontaneously grade III do not. Grade I are internal only. Both injection sclerotherapy and rubber band ligation can be used successfully for internal haemorrhoids though banding gives better results. Overall only about 5% of haemorrhoids require surgical treatment.

4. Which of the following statements on familial adenomatous polyposis (FAP) is untrue?

a) Follows an autosomal dominant inheritance pattern
b) Is more common than hereditary non-polyposis colo-rectal cancer (HNPCC)

c) Results in an almost 100% chance of colorectal malignancy
d) The underlying genetic mutation is on chromosome 5
e) Patients with FAP are at increased risk of gastric, thyroid, and adrenal tumours

[Best Answer = b]

Explanation

Mutation(s) in the adenomatous polyposis coli (APC) tumour suppressor gene on chromosome 5q leads to the development of hundreds of adenomatous polyps in early adulthood. It is usually autosomal dominant and so in most cases the patients will have one parent with the condition. Malignant transformation occurs in almost all patients by the age of 50, mandating prophylactic procto-colectomy if the patient is otherwise fit for such surgery. Patients are also at risk of developing tumours elsewhere in the GI tract. HNPCC accounts for up to 5% of colorectal cancers, FAP accounts for 1%.

5. Pseudomembranous colitis

a) Is caused by ischaemic colitis
b) Results from overgrowth of *Clostridium difficile*
c) Diagnosis is made by identification of live bacteria in stool culture
d) Is only caused by antibiotic use
e) Oral ampicillin is the treatment of choice

[Best Answer = b]

Explanation

Clostridium difficile is the most commonly identified cause of nosocomal diarrhoea in the UK. Ischaemic colitis can appear similar on colonoscopy but tend to occur in elderly arteriopaths. Symptoms are the effects of a toxin released by the bacteria, testing for this toxin not the actual bacteria is the basis of diagnosis. Most episodes follow antibiotic use, though advanced age, chemotherapy, and recent rectal surgery are also associated with pseudomembranous colitis. Treatment with oral metronidazole has been mainstay of treatment, but with the emergence of resistant strains local microbiological advice should be sought.

6. Crohn's disease

a) Usually presents in the fourth decade
b) Is caused by bovine mycobacterium
c) Most commonly affects the terminal ileum
d) Runs a more quiescent course in smokers
e) Will require surgical resection in 10% of cases

[Best Answer = c]

Explanation

Crohn's disease is an idiopathic inflammatory disease affecting the entire GI tract, but most commonly affecting the terminal ileum. It can present at any age but the peak incidence is in the second decade of life. Unlike ulcerative colitis, which is also a chronic relapsing condition, smoking is associated with a poorer prognosis and shorter periods of remission. Medical therapy is used primarily but most patients (65%) will ultimately require one or more operations.

7. Sigmoid diverticular disease

a) Prevalence is 20% in septuagenarians
b) Is premalignant
c) Can usually be diagnosed with rigid sigmoidoscopy
d) Is an indication for urgent colectomy
e) Is best treated with dietary advice in uncomplicated cases

[Best Answer = e]

Explanation

> The incidence of diverticular disease increases with age, in the UK
> > 60% will have evidence of diverticula by the age of 70. Most
> patients remain asymptomatic, but complications of the condition
> include, inflammation (diverticulitis), abscess formation, fistulation,
> bleeding, and, perforation. It is not pre-malignant. The diagnosis is
> best made at flexible endoscopy (flexible sigmoidoscopy or
> colonoscopy) or with contrast enema. As most patients are asympto-
> matic surgical excision is not indicated unless complications (above)
> arise. Most patients with mild symptoms can be treated conserva-
> tively with high fibre diets and adequate hydration.

8. Aetiological factors for sigmoid volvulus include

a) Chronic constipation
b) Low fibre diet
c) Colon cancer
d) Warfarin
e) Previous left hemi-colectomy

[Best Answer = a]

Explanation

> Volvulus of the sigmoid colon results from rotation of a floppy mobile
> colon on its relatively long mesentery. Chronic constipation or a very
> high residue diet leads to the gradual lengthening of the mesentery
> due to the weight of bowel contents. It is more common in elderly
> constipated persons and those on some psychotropic drugs which can
> interfere with bowel motility. Left hemicolectomy actually protects
> against volvulus.

9. A patient with a Dukes' C ascending colon cancer

a) Will have a poorer prognosis than a patient with Dukes' D disease
b) Can expect survival benefit with adjuvant radiotherapy
c) Is most likely to develop metastatic disease in the right kidney

d) May have any T stage using the TNM staging system

e) Should be offered post-operative radiotherapy

[Best Answer = d]

Explanation

Prognosis is better with earlier stage disease, Dukes' A being the least advanced. Chemotherapy (usually using a 5 FU) regime improves survival by 10% if given within 12 weeks of surgical excision, whereas radiotherapy has no routine place in the treatment of colonic malignancy. Using the Dukes' classification a stage C tumour is one with nodal metastases regardless of the depth of invasion in/through the bowel wall, this is one of the reasons for the increasing use of TNM staging to compare pathological stage.

10. Carcinoembryonic antigen (CEA)

a) Is not useful for clinical follow-up in colorectal cancer

b) Normal range is dependent on patient age

c) Is specific to colorectal cancers

d) May be elevated in smokers

e) Is useful as a screening test for colorectal cancer

[Best Answer = d]

Explanation

CEA is secreted by most colorectal cancer cells, but is not disease specific and may be raised in other GI malignancies (oesophagus, stomach, liver, pancreas, etc). Levels may also be elevated in patients who smoke or by chemotherapeutic agents (notably hormone modulating agents). These factors make CEA unsuitable for screening and it is best used as a follow-up tool, where by taking serial measurements upward trends can be identified.

11. Colonoscopy

a) Does not require formal mechanical bowel preparation
b) Carries a 1% perforation rate
c) Is more sensitive than Barium enema at detecting colonic polyps
d) Is safest when performed under general anaesthetic
e) Unlike ultrasound is not user dependent

[Best Answer = c]

Explanation

Successful colonoscopy requires a fully prepared bowel to allow direct inspection of the mucosa; the sensitivity of the test is reduced if preparation is not adequate. The potential complications of colonoscopy include bleeding and perforation, published perforation rates vary widely but a rate of less than one in 750 is acceptable. Colonoscopy is usually performed under "awake sedation" rather than general anaesthetic as an unconscious patient cannot complain of discomfort, which can alert the endoscopist to impending perforation. Colonoscopy should have a higher sensitivity than barium enema, but is of course highly operator dependent.

12. Anorectal (peri-anal) abscesses

a) Cause pain on defecation only
b) May discharge spontaneously into the rectum
c) Should be treated initially with high dose intra-venous antibiotics
d) Are not associated with systemic disorders
e) Are more likely to recur if a skin-derived organism is cultured

[Best Answer = b]

Explanation

Anorectal abscesses arise in the anal glands, increasing size in a confined space leads to the characteristic constant "throbbing" pain, not just pain on defecation. Abscesses may point and discharge to the skin, or into the anus or rectum. The initial treatment of all abscesses is adequate surgical drainage; antibiotics are only used if there is associated soft tissue infection. Diabetes is associated with an increased incidence of peri-anal sepsis, as is inflammatory bowel disease. The underlying organism is important as bowel-derived organisms as opposed to skin-derived organisms are associated with recurrent sepsis and the presence of an underlying fistula-in-ano.

13. Neoplastic colonic polyps include

a) Hyperplastic polyps
b) All pedunculated polyps
c) All sessile polyps
d) Inflammatory polyps
e) Adenomatous polyps

[Best Answer = e]

Explanation

The term neoplastic refers to polyps with significant malignant potential. In general these are the adenomas and polypoid carcinomas. Any polyp can be pedunculated (on a stalk) or sessile (flat). The malignant potential of adenomas depends on several factors including size, degree of dysplasia and proportion of villous architecture. Hyperplastic (metataplastic) polyps are simply areas of mucosal overgrowth. Hamartomas such as juvenile polyps consist of normal mucosal cells arranged abnormally or haphazardly.

14. Rectal prolapse

a) Delorme's procedure has a low recurrence rate
b) Always involves mucosa only
c) Banding or sclerotherapy are useful in full thickness prolapse
d) Constipation is not a recognised complication of rectopexy
e) Incontinence is an associated feature

[Best Answer = e]

Explanation

Prolapse of the rectal mucosa (partial thickness) or all layers (full thickness) is often associated with sphincter dysfunction and hence incontinence. Mucosal prolapse can be dealt with using sclerotherapy banding or simple excision; full thickness prolapse often requires more invasive surgery. Abdominal rectopexy gives the best outcome with regard to recurrence but bowel function (especially constipation) may be worsened. Per anal procedures such as Delorme's have fewer complications but a much higher recurrence rate.

15. Stomas

a) Ileostomies are mainly sited in the right lower quadrant
b) Colostomies should have a "spout" to protect the surrounding skin
c) Loop transverse colostomy is associated with fewer complications than loop ileostomy
d) Defunctioning stomas must be reversed within six months
e) Peristomal hernia usually results from ischaemia

[Best Answer = a]

Explanation

The site and type of stoma is clearly dependent on the reason for stoma formation. The consistency and nature of small bowel contents mean they are extremely irritant to skin and ileostomies are therefore spouted to keep their effluent away from skin. Defunctioning stomas (often temporary) tend to be loops and the right lower quadrant loop ileostomy has gained favour as it is simple to form and reverse and does not have the complications such as stomal prolapse associated with transverse colostomy. Defunctioning stomas should only be reversed when the anastomosis or fistula, which they are defunctioning, has healed completely. There is therefore no time limit, and indeed reversal is not always performed. A peristomal hernia may develop with a colostomy, ileostomy or urinary conduit. Factors that increase the chance of a hernia developing include obesity, increased age, and the presence of other diseases such as diabetes, chronic lung disease or cough, and poor nutritional intake. Ischaemia usually results in stenosis or retraction of the stoma.

Case Studies

Case 1

A 78-year-old man is admitted as an emergency with a four-month history of altered bowel habit, weight loss, and rectal bleeding. He has had absolute constipation for three days.

a) What is the most likely diagnosis? And why.
b) What would you expect to find on abdominal examination?
c) How would you assess the level of obstruction?
d) Is this patient likely to require fluid resuscitation? If so why?
e) What are the treatment options available to alleviate the obstruction?

Answers

a) The recent history of absolute constipation (passing neither faeces nor flatus) points to bowel obstruction, in association with the longer standing symptoms, malignancy of either colon or rectum is the most likely diagnosis.

b) Abdominal distension, resonant to percussion, with active bowel sounds. If there is significant caecal dilatation tenderness over the right colon may be present.

c) A digital rectal examination may reveal a low or mid rectal lesion, and plain abdominal X-ray may reveal an obvious "cut-off" point. The other options include flexible endoscopy, or radiography either water-soluble enema, or computer tomography (CT).

d) Yes. The patient is likely to require significant fluid resuscitation. Bowel obstruction leads to large volumes of fluid being sequestered out of the intra-vascular space and into the obstructed bowel, combined with nausea and anorexia due to obstruction. This patient is likely to be extremely unwell! They will require careful assessment and resuscitation prior to any intervention.

e) If there is complete obstruction with proximal bowel dilatation, colonic decompression is required to prevent perforation. Non-surgical decompression may be achieved using a self-expanding metallic stent placed endoscopically or radiologically. The surgical options include; primary resection of the obstructing lesion with either anastomosis or stoma formation, or if not resectable a defunctioning stoma proximal to the obstructed segment (colostomy, caecostomy, or ileostomy).

Case 2

A 27-year-old woman attends the outpatient clinic with a two-year history of altered bowel habit. She complains of intermittent abdominal bloating, "crampy" abdominal pain, and, alternating constipation and diarrhoea. Her weight is stable and she denies any per rectal bleeding.

a) What are the important differential diagnoses?
b) What investigations would you request to differentiate between these possibilities?
c) How would you manage the likely condition?
d) Are there any psychological considerations?
e) What dietary advice would you give?

Answers

a) The most likely diagnosis is irritable bowel syndrome (IBS), however inflammatory bowel diseases such as Crohns' disease or ulcerative colitis should be considered.

b) IBS should be a diagnosis of exclusion, as a "functional" disorder investigations looking at the bowel mucosa such as flexible endoscopy or barium studies will be normal, as will inflammatory markers such as C-reactive protein (CRP) or erythrocyte sedimentation rate (ESR).

c) IBS is a functional disorder and symptoms vary between patients. Treatment is therefore tailored to the patient. Often simple reassurance that there is no sinister pathology is all that is required, other treatments include anti-spasmodics (e.g. mebeverine). Dietary advice may also be of use.

d) IBS is aggravated by stress, and a careful history will often reveal an associated stressful event (house move, new job, etc.) with the onset or worsening of symptoms. There is some evidence to support the use of cognitive behavioural therapy (CBT).

e) Some patients relate symptoms to diet; this is again variable between patients. The best advice is to keep a careful food diary that can be compared to symptom severity and exclude/reduce those foods associated with symptoms. Paradoxically it is often those foods thought of as good for colonic health such as high fibre/high residue foods which irritate the colon most.

Case 3

A 22-year-old man attends the outpatient clinic concerned about his risk of developing colorectal cancer as he has a family history of the disease.

a) What is the incidence of colorectal cancer in the UK?
b) If his only family history of colon cancer is his grandfather who developed the disease at aged 87, what should you tell him?
c) What are the criteria used to diagnose hereditary non-polyposis colorectal cancer (HNPCC)?
d) What methods of screening for colorectal cancer are available? At what age would you start screening?
e) Who should be offered prophylactic colectomy?

Answers

a) The current incidence of colorectal cancer in the UK is about 60 per 100,000 per year.
b) He should be reassured that most colorectal cancers are sporadic and not related to a familial genetic predisposition. Statistically however with a single family member history his risk compared to the general population is only marginally raised (about 1.5×)
c) The "Amsterdam Criteria II" are used to identify HNPCC, they are: (1) familial adenomatous polyposis (FAP) has been excluded; (2) three or more relatives, at least one first degree with colorectal cancer; (3) two successive generations affected; (4) one colorectal Ca diagnosed before the age of 50; and (5) pathological confirmation of tumours.
d) The two methods mainly used are faecal occult blood testing, and endoscopic surveillance (flexible sigmoidoscopy or colonoscopy). The age at which screening should commence is unclear but

depends on the level of risk. Current thinking is that screening should probably begin at the age of 50, or ten years younger than the age that the youngest relative developed the disease.

e) Patients with FAP should be offered procto-colectomy, as they will all inevitably develop a colonic or rectal cancer. The other group to consider for prophylactic colectomy are those patients with long-standing total colitis as they are at significant risk of malignancy.

Case 4

A 52-year-old 40 kg woman with a 20-year history of Crohn's disease presents with symptoms suggestive of small bowel obstruction. She has had six previous laparotomies including an ileo-colic resection and four small bowel resections.

a) What are the possible causes for small bowel obstruction in this patient?
b) How would you manage this patient initially?
c) What are the consequences of multiple small bowel resections?
d) How can her nutritional status be improved?
e) What length of small bowel is required to maintain weight?

Answers

a) The two most likely causes are adhesions from previous surgery or a Crohn's stricture.

b) Initial management after full history and examination would be "drip and suck", i.e. intravenous fluid resuscitation, catheterisation, and naso-gastric tube. Temporary gut rest is often all that is needed for adhesive obstruction as spontaneous resolution is common.

c) Multiple bowel resections obviously lead to a progressively shorter gut. Ileo-colic resection and terminal ileal resections result in decreased absorption of Vitamin B12 and bile salts, and can lead to bacterial overgrowth. Eventually if enough small bowel is excised it may not be possible to absorb enough calories to maintain weight.

d) Supplements can be given as required for vitamin or mineral deficiencies, calorific support may be given in the form of high calorie or high protein drinks. Patients with a full-blown short gut syndrome may require long-term parenteral nutrition.

e) Approximately one metre of functional small bowel is considered to be the minimum for long-term weight maintenance. The length of small bowel required increases if the ileo-caecal valve is resected.

Case 5

You are asked to review a 75-year-old man with recurrent urinary tract infections, pneumaturia (the passage of air/gas bubbles in the urine), and left iliac fossa pain.

a) What diagnosis fits all these symptoms?
b) What are the possible underlying pathologies?
c) How would you investigate him further?
d) What are the other common complications of diverticular disease?
e) What is the risk of this man developing colorectal cancer?

Answers

a) The patient describes symptoms of a colo-vesical fistula, i.e. an abnormal communication between the bladder and colon.
b) The common causes of colo-vesical fistulae are malignancy (bladder or bowel), inflammatory bowel disease (Crohn's), or more often complicated diverticular disease. As the sigmoid is the site of most diverticulosis, most fistulae are from this area.
c) Investigations may include endoscopic examination of either the colon or the bladder, and radiological examinations such as CT.
d) Other presentations of complicated diverticular disease are, bleeding, diverticulitis, abscess formation, stricture, and perforation.
e) This patients' risk of developing colorectal cancer is unaffected by the presence of diverticular disease. It should always be remembered that many of the symptoms of diverticular disease are also symptoms of colonic malignancy and should therefore be investigated fully to exclude more sinister pathology.

Extended Matching Questions

EMQ 1

a. Rectal carcinoma
b. Fissure-in-ano
c. Caecal carcinoma
d. Haemorrhoids
e. Hirschprungs' disease
f. Crohns disease
g. Anal atresia
h. Sigmoid volvulus
i. Acute appendicitis

Choose the most appropriate diagnosis from the list above to fit the following scenarios:

1) A 28-year-old man presents with a three-week history of bright red rectal bleeding and a "lump" at the anal verge.
2) A 3-year-old girl is admitted with a history of painful defecation and a recent onset of constipation.
3) An 86-year-old with recurrent abdominal distension and long-term constipation.
4) A 72-year-old woman complaining of six weeks of alternating bowel habit, and a feeling of incomplete evacuation of stool.
5) A 19-year-old smoker with a three-week history of diarrhoea, colicky lower abdominal pain, and weight loss.

Answers

> **1) d.**
> Haemorrhoids typically present with fresh rectal blood. Prolapsing or external haemorrhoids are easily differentiated from condylomata and polyps by inspection and digital examination.
>
> **2) b.**
> Whilst fissure in ano is most common in young adults it can present in infancy or childhood. The associated constipation is often a result of rather than the cause of the fissure.

EMQ 2

a. End ileostomy
b. Loop ileostomy
c. End colostomy and mucous fistula
d. Loop colostomy
e. Ileal conduit
f. Hartmann's procedure
g. Gastrostomy
h. Ileal pouch

Which of the above stomas would best suit the following cases?

1) A 76-year-old man awaiting long course pre-operative radiotherapy. He has an obstructing low rectal carcinoma, and a competent ileo-caecal valve.
2) A 52-year-old woman (who does not wish to undergo colectomy) with chronic constipation resulting in a mega-colon.
3) A 25-year-old man undergoing a restorative procto-colectomy (pouch procedure) for ulcerative colitis.
4) A 62-year-old man taken back to theatre having developed a complete anastomotic dehiscence and peritonitis seven days following a left hemi-colectomy.
5) A patient undergoing a pan procto colectomy.

Answers

1) d.
This patient needs colonic decompression while he undergoes radio-therapy. If the lesion is too low to be stented a stoma above the level of obstruction will be required. If the ileo-caecal valve is competent, a loop ileostomy will not decompress the colon and a loop colostomy in sigmoid or transverse colon is the best option.

2) b.
A loop ileostomy is the best option from the list above. Another option is a procedure called an ante-grade continent enema, this uses the appendix as a conduit to allow the colon to be irrigated periodi-cally. It is used in both adults and children.

3) b.
It is usual to de-function the bowel in these patients to allow the pouch and the pouch-anal anastomosis to mature and heal. As the procedure involves a total colectomy, loop ileostomy is the only option.

4) c.
In cases of anastomotic leak with faecal spillage it is not safe to per-form another primary anastomosis and an end colostomy should be formed, the rectal stump may also be brought out as a mucus fistula.

5) a.
This operation removes the entire large bowel and the anal canal. The terminal ileum is used to form the stoma.

EMQ 3

a. Colonoscopy
b. Barium enema
c. Flexible sigmoidoscopy
d. Chest X-ray
e. Mesenteric angiography
f. Ultrasound scan of abdomen
g. CT scan of chest abdomen and pelvis
h. Gastroscopy

Choose the most appropriate investigation for each scenario:

1) An asymptomatic 72-year-old man with iron deficiency anaemia and a positive faecal occult blood test. Colonoscopy has been normal.
2) A 48-year-old man with biopsy proven mid rectal cancer.
3) An 88-year-old woman with torrential rectal bleeding. Both gastroscopy and colonoscopy have failed to reveal the cause.
4) A 21-year-old man whose father and paternal aunt were diagnosed with colorectal cancer in their 40s.
5) A 30-year-old woman with bright red rectal bleeding on defecation and no obvious anal canal abnormality.

Answers

1) h.
FOB does not differentiate between upper and lower GI blood loss therefore both gastroscopy and colonoscopy should be performed.

2) g.
CT is used for staging local disease and to identify any metastatic disease. MRI gives more detail of local invasion and may help determine the need for pre-operative radiotherapy. Colonoscopy is the best modality for assessing the proximal colon to exclude other primary (synchronous) tumours.

3) e.
An attempt at colonoscopy is worthwhile but views are often poor due to blood in the lumen of the bowel. In this desperate situation, with active bleeding, mesenteric angiography may reveal the bleeding point. A likely diagnosis in this age group is bleeding from either angiodysplasia of the colon or from diverticular disease.

4) a.
Such a strong family history is an indication for screening colonoscopy, referral to a clinical geneticist should be considered.

5) c.
Bright red rectal bleeding usually arises in the rectum or distal sigmoid, it is therefore appropriate to perform a flexible sigmoidoscopy, if however no pathology is found the rest of the colon should be imaged.

EMQ 4

a. Biofeedback therapy
b. Colostomy
c. Lateral internal sphincterotomy
d. Haemorrhoidectomy
e. Biofeedback therapy
f. Delorme's procedure
g. Abdominal rectopexy

Choose the most appropriate treatment for each scenario:

1) A 35-year-old male with an anterior midline anal fissure who has failed topical therapy.
2) A 40-year-old female with a three-year history of constipation. Defaecating proctography shows failure to relax the puborectalis muscle and inability to evacuate the rectum.
3) A 45-year-old female with good medical health with a full thickness rectal prolapse on straining.
4) A 70-year-old female complains of tenesmus and the passage of mucus PR. On examination she has a full thickness rectal prolapse. She is otherwise well.
5) A 46-year-old man with painful bleeding haemorrhoids, which prolapse on defaecation and require manual reduction.

Answers

1) c.
Initial treatment of anal fissures consists of stool softeners and topical cream such as 2% Diltiazem or 0.2% GTN paste. If the patient remains symptomatic treatment is aimed at temporary or permanent relaxation of the internal anal sphincter by means of either botulinum toxin injection or lateral internal sphincterotomy (= surgical division of the sphincter).

2) a.
Longstanding constipation is usually the result of slow colonic transit or failure to evacuate the rectum due to pelvic floor dysfunction. Failure of relaxation of the puborectalis muscle can be demonstrated by defaecating proctography and usually responds to biofeedback therapy.

3) g.

Full thickness rectal prolapse is best treated surgically using an abdominal or perineal approach. In an otherwise healthy patient the abdominal approach offers the best chance of success with low rates of recurrence. Mobilisation and fixation of the rectum is performed by using the open or laparoscopic approach with or without simultaneous resection of the sigmoid colon. In unfit patients the Delorme's procedure is an alternative.

4) f.

In an elderly patient symptomatic partial thickness rectal prolapse is sometimes correctable by means of rubber band ligation via a proctoscope. This can be performed in the outpatient or endoscopy unit. If this fails and the patient is fit for general anaesthesia, a Delorme's procedure can be performed. This consists of excision of the prolapsing mucosa with plication of the underlying tissues.

5) d.

Patients with third degree haemorrhoids (i.e. those requiring manual reduction) are not suitable for rubber band ligation or injection schlerotherapy. Operative haemorrhoidectomy may be performed using open, closed, or stapled techniques.

EMQ 5

a. Colonic stent
b. Pre-operative chemoradiotherapy
c. Post-operative radiotherapy
d. Post-operative chemotherapy
e. Radiofrequency ablation
f. Defunctioning stoma
g. Total mesorectal excision
h. Intra-operative radiotherapy

Choose the most appropriate treatment for the following patients:

1) A 70-year-old male with multiple co-morbidities presents with an obstructing sigmoid cancer. CT scan shows multiple metastases in the liver and lungs.
2) A 35-year-old male presents with low rectal cancer. MRI suggests possible prostatic invasion.

3) A 40-year-old female is two weeks post-anterior resection for rectal cancer. Histology confirms a T3 adenocarcinoma. Circumferential resection margins are 2 mm. Two of 20 lymph nodes are positive for metastatic adenocarcinoma.
4) A 60-year-old male presents with a mid rectal cancer. Staging MRI suggests a T2 N1 lesion. The patient is otherwise well.
5) A 70-year-old male patient presents with an obstructing low rectal cancer. He has multiple medical co-morbidities and is considered unfit for major surgery.

Answers

1) a.
The best form of palliation for this patient would be insertion of an endoluminal metallic stent to relieve the obstruction. This can be inserted either endoscopically or radiologically. Should stent insertion not be possible then a defunctioning stoma proximal to the sigmoid would suffice. Referral to an oncologist should then be performed to consider palliative chemotherapy.

2) b.
Locally advanced rectal tumour should be initially treated with a five-week course of pre-operative radiotherapy. The addition of chemotherapy pre-operatively will improve response rates should the patient's medical condition allow. Restaging by means of CT or MRI should then be performed prior to considering the patient suitable for surgical intervention.

3) d.
Circumferential resection margins of greater than 1 mm are considered adequate for tumour clearance. Referral to an oncologist to consider adjuvant chemotherapy should be performed in the presence of any lymph nodes positive for adenocarcinoma.

4) g.
Cross-sectional imaging has revealed a tumour with surrounding lymph nodes which can be completely resected by means of a total mesorectal excision. There is no indication for down staging by means of long course radiotherapy prior to surgical resection. There is a growing body of evidence however which suggests that a short

(five-day) course of radiotherapy prior to surgery may improve rates of local recurrence. Repeat staging prior to surgery is not necessary in these patients.

5) f.
Relief of obstruction by means of a defunctioning stoma is the most appropriate treatment in these circumstances. Endoluminal stent insertion for a rectal tumour, which is digitally palpable, would result in an unacceptable degree of tenesmus. Palliative radiotherapy or medical optimisation can then be considered.

Chapter 5   The Acute Abdomen

Klaus Overbeck and Dorota Overbeck-Zubrzycka

Multiple Choice Questions

[Each single best answer (SBA) question comprises a stem and a number of answers. You are asked to decide which single item represents the best answer to the question.]

1. Abdominal pain

A 48-year-old man is brought by ambulance with severe abdominal pain. He is a heavy smoker and drinks approximately two bottles of wine per day. His amylase is found to be 920. You diagnose acute pancreatitis. Which of the following systems are not used for staging the severity of this condition?

    a) APACHE II
    b) CRP
    c) Glasgow criteria
    d) Gleason system
    e) Ranson's score

[Best Answer = d]

Explanation

> They are many clinical systems used to assess the severity of acute pancreatitis and to predict the prognosis of this condition. These include the Ranson criteria, Glasgow criteria, and acute physiology and chronic health evaluation (APACHE II) criteria. CRP is also an important prognostic marker of acute pancreatitis. Gleason scoring is used in prostate cancer.

2. Upper GI bleeding

A 37-year-old factory worker presents to the A&E with haematemesis. He has epigastric pain that has been present for the last three months. On examination, he has gynaecomastia and spider naevi and admits to a heavy intake of alcohol. The following might typically be seen in this type of patient:

a) Melena
b) Low serum urea
c) Hypochromic macrocytic anaemia
d) Hyperchromic microcytic anaemia
e) High platelet count

[Best Answer = a]

Explanation

Patients with alcohol-induced liver cirrhosis can develop portal hypertension. This can in turn cause oesophageal varices. Bleeding from oesophageal varices is common in these patients and once altered in the GI tract presents with melena. Chronic loss of blood from the digestive tract results in hypochromic, microcytic anaemia. Serum urea tends to rise in significant GI bleeding due to absorption of proteins from the GI tract.

3. Abdominal pain

A 71-year-old man, a heavy smoker with a history of hypertension, is brought by ambulance after having collapsed in the street. He is complaining of abdominal pain radiating to his back and is severely hypotensive. Which of the following is the most appropriate next step in management?

a) Angiography
b) CT scan
c) Endoscopy
d) Laparotomy
e) Ultrasonography

[Best Answer = d]

Explanation

This is probably a ruptured aneurysm. In patients over 50 years of age with a collapse associated with abdominal or back pain assume rupture of abdominal aortic aneurysm until proven otherwise. Such cases should be taken immediately to theatre without delay for investigations. There is no need for any diagnostic imaging. He needs to go to theatre.

4. Child with acute abdomen

A ten-year-old boy with a five-hour history of periumbilical pain presents with severe right lower quadrant pain, nausea and vomiting. He has not eaten the whole day. He even refuses his favourite ice creams. Which diagnosis is most likely?

a) Acute appendicitis
b) Constipation
c) Inflammatory bowel disease
d) Mesenteric adenitis
e) Meckel's diverticulitis

[Best Answer = a]

Explanation

The most likely diagnosis is acute appendicitis. In children this can be difficult to diagnose. Typically there is pain and tenderness in the right iliac fossa combined with loss of appetite, nausea or vomiting. The vomiting with appendicitis is usually single or few times as opposed to the frequent vomiting found in gastroenteritis. Equally diarrhoea is not typical for appendicitis unless a pelvic abscess has formed which irritates the rectum. Other possibilities include mesenteric adenitis and Meckels diverticulitis.

5. Abdominal pain

A 41-year-old man is admitted with severe abdominal pain for the last ten hours. It started in the upper part of his abdomen and has later become generalised. He has vomited twice. Normally very loud and talkative, he is now lying very still, quiet, avoiding any movements. What is the very first thing you should do when assessing the patient?

a) 100% oxygen mask
b) Analgesia
c) Assess his airway

d) Check blood pressure

e) Insert a large bore IV cannula

[Best Answer = c]

Explanation

> Mnemonic for accessing any ill patient is ABCDE: airway, breathing, circulation, disability and exposure. An obstructed airway is the most immediate threats to life. To assess a patients airway ask him a question; for example, ask how he is feeling. If the patient responds verbally, he has an intact airway and is breathing adequately. The next step is assessment of the circulation and securing IV access.

6. Abdominal pain

While walking his dog in the morning a 36-year-old man experiences sudden excruciating pain in his right flank and back which radiates into his right groin. Which of the following is the most likely diagnosis?

a) Acute mesenteric ischaemia

b) Muscle spasm

c) Ureteric colic

d) Prolapsed intervertebral disc

e) Ruptured abdominal aortic aneurysm

[Best Answer = c]

Explanation

> Lifetime risk of developing a ureteric stone is about 5% and 30- to 60-year-old men are most commonly affected. Ureteric colic typically causes severe colicky loin to groin pain. It may radiate into the scrotum in men and the labia in women. It may also cause frequency, urgency and dysuria. Microscopic haematuria nearly always accompanies the pain in ureteric colic.

7. Abdominal pain

A 45-year-old woman with long-standing rheumatoid arthritis presents following the sudden onset of severe epigastric pain. She lies very still and breathes shallowly. What is the most likely diagnosis?

a) Acute cholecystitis
b) Acute pancreatitis
c) Indigestion
d) Myocardial infarction
e) Perforated peptic ulcer

[Best Answer = e]

Explanation

> The presentation is very suggestive of a duodenal ulcer with perforation. The onset of pain is sudden and intensifies to the maximum. Patients usually remember exactly what they were doing when the pain started. They typically avoid movements.

8. Abdominal pain

An 18-year-old girl attends with lower abdominal pain. She is well and has a temperature of 37.7°C. Her last period was six weeks ago, but she has irregular cycles. Since it is after midnight you decide to observe her overnight. What should you do before sending her to the ward?

a) Chest X-ray
b) Full blood count
c) Pregnancy test
d) Urine bacteriology
e) Ultrasound

[Best Answer = c]

Explanation

> This patient may simply have UTI but may also have appendicitis. All fertile women with lower abdominal pain may have an ectopic pregnancy and this always needs to be excluded on first assessment. A urine dipstix should be performed in A&E and if abnormal should be sent for culture, although the bacteriology would take 24 to 48 hours to get a result. It is not wrong to do a full blood count but it is not required as an emergency test after midnight as it will not alter the management, which is observation and review.

9. Abdominal pain

A 15-year-old student complains of crampy abdominal pain accompanied by diarrhoea with blood and mucous. He has been recently diagnosed as having ankylosing spondylitis. Choose the most likely diagnosis.

    a) Inflammatory bowel disease
    b) Gastroenteritis
    c) Irritable bowel syndrome
    d) Meckel's diverticulitis
    e) Necrotising enterocolitis

[Best Answer = a]

Explanation

An acute episode of inflammatory bowel disease presents with abdominal pain, diarrhoea, passage of blood and mucous per rectum. Inflammatory bowel disease is associated with ankylosing spondylitis — an inflammatory disease of the spine or sacro-iliac joints.

10. Intestinal obstruction

A 59-year-old bank executive is admitted with abdominal distension, vomiting and absolute constipation. You order an abdominal X-ray. Which of the following features would make you think that you are dealing with small bowel obstruction?

    a) Central position of distended loops
    b) Dilated bowel with haustrae
    c) Peripheral position of distended loops
    d) Presence of air in the rectum
    e) Haustra crossing the bowel width

[Best Answer = a]

Explanation

> X-rays of the abdomen are important in diagnosing the presence of small bowel obstruction. When obstruction occurs, both fluid and gas collect in the intestine. They produce a characteristic pattern called "air-fluid levels". The more distal the obstruction is, the more numerous the gas-fluid levels. Distended small bowel loops are positioned in the centre of the abdomen. Characteristically, valvulae coniventes (seen in the small bowel) completely cross the bowel width, whereas haustra (seen in the large bowel) only partially cross the lumen.

11. Intestinal obstruction

A 70-year-old nursing home resident is admitted with suspected bowel obstruction. On examination his abdomen is grossly distended but soft and non-tender to palpation. On the basis of abdominal X-ray the diagnosis of colonic pseudo-obstruction is made. The following are true for this condition:

a) Increased bowel sounds are usually present
b) Colonic pseudo-obstruction does not cause a perforation
c) Colonic pseudo-obstruction is characterised by early vomiting
d) Diarrhoea makes colonic pseudo-obstruction unlikely
e) Opiate analgesia is not indicated as it may mask acute abdominal signs

[Best Answer = d]

Explanation

> Colonic pseudo-obstruction is a functional disorder with the signs and symptoms of an acute large bowel obstruction but no evidence of mechanical obstruction. It affects most commonly the mentally impaired, elderly and hospitalised patients. The colon may become massively dilated and if not decompressed perforation may occur. The presenting complaint is massive abdominal distension which may be associated with abdominal pain, nausea and vomiting.

12. Child with acute abdomen

A tearful three-year-old boy is brought in by his mum. He has intermittent abdominal pain but looks well. The mother tells you he has not moved his bowels for the last three days. His abdomen looks slightly distended but is not tender when you distract him. He is apyrexial. Choose the most likely diagnosis.

a) Constipation
b) Incarcerated hernia
c) Irritable bowel syndrome
d) Meckel's diverticulitis
e) Necrotising enterocolitis

[Best Answer = a]

Explanation

> Constipation in children is a common complaint. In most cases it is functional probably because the child has been avoiding moving their bowels due to "toilet training" attempts by the parents, stress or simply being too busy playing. The stool then hardens due to further absorption of water and defecation becomes painful which leads to further reluctance. Treatment consists initially of enemas or oral laxatives but dietary and behaviour change are also important.

13. Abdominal mass

A previously fit and well 77-year-old lady comes to her GP with generalised abdominal discomfort, distension and weight loss. Since yesterday she has been short of breath. She has never had children, neither has she ever taken the contraceptive pill. On examination a large hard abdominal mass is palpable below the umbilicus arising from the pelvis. Which of the following are not associated with the underlying condition?

a) BRCA receptor +ve
b) Early menarche
c) Late menopause
d) Late menarche
e) Late menopause

[Best Answer = d]

Explanation

This woman is likely to have advanced ovarian cancer. The signs and symptoms of ovarian cancer are non-specific and patients present late. Abdominal pain, vaginal bleeding, bloating, distension, irregular menses, change in bowel habits are found. Risk factors associated with ovarian cancer are effectively prolonged exposure to oestrogens and hence nulliparity, early menarche, late menopause, history of breast cancer and HRT.

14. Jaundice

A 25-year-old woman with a two-year history of intermittent upper abdominal pain has developed jaundice and rigours. She tells you that her doctor in another hospital has "cleaned out the liver with a camera last year" and that she is on a waiting list to have her gallbladder removed. Which of these tests is most appropriate to confirm the diagnosis?

a) Laparoscopy
b) Liver function tests
c) ERCP
d) Serum amylase
e) Ultrasound

[Best Answer = e]

Explanation

This patient is likely to have a stone in the bile duct. This may cause infection of the bile ducts known as cholangitis. If the bile ducts are obstructed, an ultrasound will show that but may also show gallstones in the ducts. Treatment consists of intravenous antibiotics and decompression of the bile ducts by removing the obstruction. The patient in this scenario has previously undergone an ERCP. She still may have some stones left in her bile ducts. Liver function tests should also be performed to look for an obstructive picture and an amylase should be sent to exclude pancreatitis.

15. Acute abdomen post-operatively

A 70-year-old retired engineer underwent a right hemi-colectomy for a carcinoma. His recovery is complicated by a myocardial infarct and pneumonia, for which he has been receiving antibiotics. You are called three days post-operatively because of increasing abdominal distension. He is on a ventilator with a nasogastric tube and can provide no history. He has no bowel sounds and his abdomen is soft. A plain abdominal X-ray reveals dilated small and large bowel loops. Which of the following diagnoses can be ruled out?

a) An anastomotic leak
b) Paralytic ileus
c) Acute gastric dilatation
d) Colonic pseudo-obstruction
e) Appendicitis

[Best Answer = e]

Explanation

A post-operative ileus is probably the most likely cause but it could be an early anastomotic leak and less likely colonic pseudo-obstruction. Anastomotic leak should be considered whenever there is unexplained post-operative deterioration. Acute gastric dilatation is a dangerous complication which can occur after surgery or trauma. Hiccoughs or vomiting, rising pulse and shock may occur. Treatment is insertion of a nasogastric tube but it is less likely here since the patient already has a nasogastric tube and the distension involves small and large bowel on the X-ray. By definition a right hemicolectomy involves removal of the appendix and so appendicitis can be ruled out.

Case Studies

Case 1

A 21-year-old postman attends the A&E department at 2am with abdominal pain. It started 24 hours ago around the umbilicus. Two hours ago it has shifted to the right iliac fossa. The pain is constant in nature. The patient has vomited clear fluid once and had mildly loose stools about five hours ago. He is pyrexial (38.2°C). On examination, there is tenderness on deep palpation over the right iliac fossa, but no guarding or rebound tenderness.

a) What is the most likely diagnosis?
b) What differential diagnoses would you consider in this case?
c) Why has the pain shifted from the central region to the right iliac fossa?
d) What investigations should be carried out?
e) Is analgesia indicated?
f) What is the treatment?

Answers

a) Acute appendicitis.
b) Differential diagnoses: There are many! The following are the most common.

- Renal tract stone
- Urinary tract infection
- Meckel's diverticulitis
- Mesenteric adenitis
- Testicular torsion
- Crohn's disease
- Internal hernia.

c) Initially, patients with appendicitis classically present with visceral, vague, poorly localised, periumbilical pain (due to inflammation and distension of the wall of the appendix). Within six to 48 hours, the pain becomes localised in the right iliac fossa as the local parietal peritoneum becomes inflamed (somatic pain).

d) Investigations:
- Urinanalysis
- Full blood count, urea and electrolytes, CRP may be helpful, but in the decision to operate is usually made on clinical grounds.
- Imaging (such as an ultrasound) is not routinely indicated unless the diagnosis is uncertain.

e) Analgesia

Analgesia should be given to patients with acute abdominal pain if required. Opiates in appropriate doses do not mask the clinical findings of the abdominal examination and can make the examination more meaningful.

f) Treatment:

Antibiotic treatment is not indicated unless the decision is made to operate since it may mask the symptoms and the rate of recurrence is high. If the patient is not too unwell, the operation can often be safely deferred until the morning. The patient should be kept nil by mouth and started on I.V. fluids. The surgery is appendicectomy.

Case 2

A 27-year-old fishmonger has just finished working a very busy shift. He starts to complain of pain in his left flank, which suddenly becomes intense and radiates into his left groin and testes. He feels sick, and vomits repeatedly. The pain becomes so severe that he is writhing in agony on his bed. His abdomen is soft, with no tenderness or guarding. Routine analysis of his urine shows 2 + blood, 1 + ketones, and 1 + protein.

a) What is the most likely diagnosis?
b) What are the possible underlying causes?
c) What radiological investigations should be carried out?
d) What is the management of his condition?
e) What is a staghorn calculus?

Answers

a) Acute renal colic.
b) Causes:

- Dehydration with reduced urine output
- Increased protein intake

- Heavy physical exercise
- Use of drugs associated with stone formation.

c) Radiological investigations:

- Plain abdominal X-ray (KUB = kidneys, ureters, bladder).
- Intravenous urography (IVU)
- Non-contrast CT scan
- Ultrasound.

d) Management:
Most small ureteric stones pass spontaneously and the patient is advised to drink plenty to ease this process. About 15%–20% of patients require invasive intervention due to stone size, continued obstruction, infection, or intractable pain. Techniques used include: extracorporeal shock wave lithotripsy (ESWL), ureteroscopy, percutaneous nephrolithotomy, and open nephrostomy.

e) A staghorn calculus
It is a stone that has grown to the shape of the renal pelvis and fills the calices of the kidney. It is caused by urease-producing bacteria like Proteus.

Case 3

Following the marriage of his daughter, an elderly man is brought into the hospital by an ambulance. He has been complaining of lower abdominal pain. The patient has also noticed some urinary hesitancy, nocturia and poor stream of micturation for a year. His pulse is 120/min and blood pressure 130/90. On examination you can feel a large tender mass in his lower abdomen which is dull to percussion.

a) What is the most likely diagnosis?
b) How should the patient be managed initially?
c) Should the patient be referred to a specialist team? Explain your answer.
d) What is the importance of intravenous fluid therapy?
e) What further investigations are required?

Answers

a) Urinary retention.
b) Transurethral catheterisation.

c) Yes — the urology team. The patient is likely to require further investigations and treatment.

d) Patients with urinary retention have often a degree of post-renal failure and once flow is restored the patient may become polyuric and pass large amounts of urine which needs replacing with fluids.

e) An ultrasound of the urinary tract and the prostate as well. Some feel that a PSA should also be requested since the cause of the retention could be a prostate carcinoma. Others argue that catheterisation and rectal examination can push up the PSA and that this should therefore not be carried out in the acute setting.

Case 4

A 55-year-old unemployed female is admitted with abdominal pain to a surgical ward. She has admitted to chronic alcohol dependence. The pain started quite suddenly eight hours ago and since then she has vomited five times. The patient describes the pain as being severe and radiating round both sides to her back. She prefers sitting forward. On examination the patient is thin, looks unwell, but has no signs of jaundice or anaemia. She is tender in the epigastrium and guarding is noted, with scanty bowel sounds. Initial observations reveal a pulse of 117/minute and a blood pressure of 115/67.

a) What is the most likely diagnosis?
b) What is the differential diagnosis?
c) Name possible aetiological factors of the underlying condition.
d) What are the complications of this condition?
e) What investigations should be carried out?
f) What is the management of her condition?
g) What are the indications for surgery?

Answers

a) Acute pancreatitis.
b) Differential diagnosis: There are many! These are the most common.

- Biliary colic, cholangitis, cholecystitis
- Chronic pancreatitis
- Duodenal ulcer, acute gastritis, gastric ulcer

- Diverticulitis
- Myocardial infarction.

c) Causes. Again there are many.

- Alcohol and gallstones are the most common.

d) Complications can be systemic or local. For example:
Systemic complications:

- Multiorgan failure due to SIRS
- Diabetes.

Local complications:

- Abdominal fluid collections, cysts and abscesses
- Bleeding.

e) Investigations:

- Full blood count, U&E, liver function test, serum calcium
- Amylase and lipase
- Arterial blood gas
- Chest X-ray
- CT abdomen.

f) Management:

Treatment is supportive with I.V. fluids and analgesia and oxygen if needed. If severe or complicated, antibiotics and treatment of complications will be required. In very severe cases this will require management on an intensive care unit.

g) Indications for surgery:

- Infected pancreatic necrosis
- Abscess formation
- Bleeding.

Case 5

A 77-year-old male is brought to the hospital. His wife reports that he has complained of central abdominal pain for the past 24 hours, which has become more generalised and is worsening. On examination, the patient appears to be confused, with a blood pressure of 95/55 and a pulse of 105/minute. The abdomen is distended, diffusely tender and the patient has marked rebound tenderness. He has a history of atrial fibrillation and is diabetic. His WBC is 33,000 and the lactate 8 mmol/l.

a) What is the most likely diagnoses?
b) How should the patient be managed initially?
c) What investigations should be performed?
d) Why is he hypotensive?
e) What are the common causes of bowel ischaemia?

Answers

a) The patient has generalised peritonitis. The patient could have perforated diverticular disease but may also have mesenteric ischaemia. This condition is most commonly caused by an embolus of cardiac origin which occludes the superior mesenteric artery. This vessel supplies the small bowel and colon up to the splenic flexure. The occlusion causes severe pain initially leading to peritonitis when the gangrenous bowel perforates.

b) This patient is in hypovolaemic shock and likely to be severely fluid depleted. Therefore, the first priority is to restore his circulating volume. The patient's only chance of survival is an urgent laparotomy but the severity of his illness and the presence of diffuse peritonitis are ominous signs.

c) There is no need to perform any diagnostic imaging in this situation. The investigations should be focused on resuscitation so the blood cross-match, urea, electrolytes and the full blood count are relevant.

d) Ischaemia of the gut due to a mesenteric infarct leads to perforation and peritonitis. This is the cause of dehydration since intravascular fluid depletion develops rapidly due to third space loss (the bowel) and sepsis. Characteristic findings in mesenteric ischaemia are high WBC and acidosis.

e) Aetiology:
Arterial — occlusive

- Cardiac arrhythmias, particularly atrial fibrillation causing emboli
- Recent myocardial infarction again causing emboli
- Atherosclerosis leading to thrombotic occlusion of a vessel.

Arterial — non-occlusive

- Hypotension in severe illness or congestive heart failure
- Following CABG (may also be embolic)

Venous obstruction

- Thrombophilia
- Secondary due to malignancy, compression and local inflammation, e.g. pancreatitis.

Extended Matching Questions

EMQ 1

Diagnosis of acute upper abdominal pain

a. Abdominal aortic aneurysm
b. Epigastric hernia
c. Acute cholangitis
d. Acute cholecystitis
e. Acute pancreatitis
f. Lower lobe pneumonia
g. Mesenteric ischaemia
h. Myocardial infarction
i. Perforated oesophagus
j. Perforated peptic ulcer

For each patient with upper abdominal pain, select the single most likely diagnosis:

1) A 25-year-old office worker, a heavy smoker with a long history of dyspepsia, presents with a five-hour history of sudden onset upper abdominal pain. Pain is constant, severe, aggravated by movement and coughing. He is sweaty and clammy and his abdomen is rigid on examination. His heart rate is 150/min.

2) A 30-year-old obese woman presents with a two-day history of right upper quadrant pain, which has worsened over the last seven hours. She has a temperature of 38°C and is complaining of nausea. She has vomitted twice.

3) A 50-year-old man, with a history of alcohol abuse in the past, presents with epigastric pain and vomiting. The pain started suddenly one day after a party at work and it radiates into his back. He looks unwell and his abdomen is tender in the epigastrium, but soft.

4) A 55-year-old man is admitted with a four-hour history of acute epigastric pain, shortness of breath, chest tightness, heaviness and nausea but not vomiting. He gets angina occasionally.

5) An obese male complains of severe epigastric pains and tells you that he can feel a lump in his abdominal wall halfway between the xyphoid and the umbilicus. He is otherwise well.

Answers

1) j.
Peptic ulcers are more common in men and in smokers. A history of indigestion is commonly found. Sudden onset of severe, acute constant pain aggravated by movement is typical for an intestinal perforation. The intensity depends on what type of content is leaking into the abdominal cavity. Gastric acid causes intense chemical irritation leading to immediate pain and guarding. The rigidity of the abdomen is typical. A tachycardia is an important finding indicating severe pain and is a part of the septic picture.

2) d.
Cholecystitis is an inflammation of the gallbladder caused commonly by gallstones obstructing the gallbladder outflow leading to stasis and inflammation due to infection of the bile. Initially symptoms are localised to the right upper quadrant.

3) e.
Over 80% cases of pancreatitis are caused by high alcohol intake or gallstones. The pancreas is a retroperitoneal organ, localised behind the stomach, where it forms a part of the posterior wall of the lesser sack. Symptoms from pancreatitis are therefore typically back and epigastric pain.

4) h.
An acute inferior myocardial infarct due to a thrombosis of the right coronary artery can cause upper abdominal pain and nausea. Therefore, make sure that any patient with upper abdominal pain has an ECG.

5) b.
Epigastric hernias are caused by a weakness of the linea alba between the rectus muscles. Most epigastric hernias are harmless since they contain only pre-peritoneal fat or a small amount of omentum. However, if large they may contain bowel, stomach or even liver. Obese men are commonly affected.

EMQ 2

Diagnosis of acute central abdominal pain

a. Acute appendicitis
b. Acute pancreatitis
c. Diverticulitis
d. Intestinal obstruction
e. Intestinal pseudo-obstruction
f. Irritable bowel syndrome
g. Mesenteric ischaemia
h. Ruptured abdominal aortic aneurysm
i. Testicular torsion
j. Ovarian cyst rupture

For each patient with central abdominal pain, select the single most likely diagnosis:

1) A 67-year-old retired man presents with an increasing abdominal distension for four days. He has intermittent griping abdominal pain. He moved his bowels a week ago and has not passed any wind for three days. Two hours ago, he vomited copiously twice.

2) A 75-year-old lady presents to the emergency department with a history of severe central abdominal pain, which has lasted for two hours and then got better. She has uncontrolled atrial fibrillation. Her abdomen is mildly tender but she looks very unwell. While you examine her, the pain is worsening again. Her arterial blood gasses show a pH of 7.21 and her serum lactate is 5 mmol/l.

3) A 78-year-old retired man with a history of smoking and hypertension has developed sudden severe pain in his back and abdomen. His blood pressure is 120/70 mmHg and the pulse rate 110/min. Whilst you are talking to him, he becomes obtunded and his blood pressure drops to 65 mmHg systolic.

4) A 35-year-old female comes to the outpatient clinic. She appears stressed and is complaining of severe abdominal pains for years. This time the pain is worse than it has ever been. Whenever she eats the food "moves right through her". Her bowels move irregularly. The abdomen is vaguely tender.

5) A 95-year-old nursing home resident with a history of dementia is admitted with gross abdominal distension. Her abdomen is tympanic, not tender and the rectum is empty. The abdominal X-ray shows a distended colon up to the splenic flexure and there is gas in the rectum.

Answers

1) d.

The main features of intestinal obstruction are distension, vomitting, colicky pain and absolute constipation. Like any hollow tube, the bowel can be obstructed by compression from outside (adhesions, strangulated hernias), because of a mass in the wall (colonic cancer) or be blocked by something inside the tube (polyps).

2) g.

Acute mesenteric ischaemia is one of the most lethal abdominal emergencies with mortality of 80%. The reason is the apparent lack of symptoms until the bowel has already infarcted. The patient typically experiences intense pain when the infarct occurs but it eases off until the bowel perforates. Characteristically, patients look more unwell than clinical signs suggest. Therefore, you must have a high index of suspicion. Mesenteric ischaemia often affects older patients, especially those with atrial fibrillation or atherosclerotic disease. Typically, white cell count and serum lactate are high at an early stage.

3) h.

Rupture of a abdominal aortic aneurysm leads to death unless the patient undergoes urgent repair of the aneurysm. The aorta is a retroperitoneal organ so commonly ruptured aneurysms cause a back pain. Usually you will be able to feel a pulsatile mass in the abdomen.

4) f.

Irritable bowel syndrome (IBS) is a functional disorder of the bowel. Many of the symptoms are similar to those of GI malignancies. So the diagnosis of IBS can only be made if all other possible causes are excluded (including inflammatory bowel disease). The presentation is with abdominal pain, change in the bowel habits, flatulence, tenesmus and abdominal bloating.

5) e.

Colonic pseudo obstruction is mostly found in elderly, hospitalised patients often with a mental illness like dementia but also patients after gynaecological or orthopaedic operations. The underlying pathology is poorly understood but colonic dysmobilty is found causing air trapping but no mechanical obstruction. The patient is at risk of a perforation if left untreated.

EMQ 3

Diagnosis of acute lower abdominal pain
a. Acute appendicitis
b. Colonic cancer
c. Diverticulitis
d. Intestinal obstruction
e. Mittelschmerz
f. Ovarian cyst torsion
g. Pelvic inflammatory disease
h. Ruptured ectopic pregnancy
i. Testicular torsion
j. Ureteric colic

For each patient with lower abdominal pain, select the single most likely diagnosis:

1) An 18-year-old student presents with abdominal pain, which started the day before. Initially the pain was central and the patient thought it was "just a trapped wind". However, since this morning the pain is in the right iliac fossa. He walks bent over and prefers lying down on the left side with the knees drawn up to the chest.

2) A 28-year-old woman complains of sudden onset suprapubic pain. It started one hour ago. Her last period finished ten days ago and the pregnancy test is negative.

3) A 76-year-old woman presents with lower abdominal pain lasting for the last three days. Pain is progressive in nature and accompanied by abdominal distension and vomitting. She does not remember when she last moved her bowels. Her past medical history includes a laparotomy for ovarian cancer six weeks ago.

4) A 16-year-old student is woken suddenly at night with severe testicular and lower abdominal pain radiating to his groin. Urinalysis is negative.

5) Sixteen hours ago a 59-year-old housewife developed left lower quadrant abdominal pain, which is constant, severe and deep. Last year she had a few episodes of colicky, diffuse abdominal pain accompanied by constipation and diarrhoea.

Answers

1) a.

Appendicitis presents with abdominal pain, tenderness, vomitting and fever. Initially, the pain, caused by the inflammation of the appendix, is poorly localised in the centre of the abdomen. Once the appendicitis has caused inflammation of the adjacent peritoneum, the pain is felt in the right iliac fossa. This shift of pain is typical for appendicitis although not always present. Bending the hip reduces the tension on the inflamed peritoneum and is therefore more comfortable.

2) e.

Mittelschmerz is the German word for painful ovulation (Mittel = middle and Schmerz = pain — "pain in the middle of cycle"). The pain can be similar to the pain in appendicitis. It lasts from few hours to two to three days. It is one sided and affects up to 20% of women. It is caused by the stretched capsule of the ovary when a follicle ruptures or by the contents of the ruptured follicle irritating the peritoneum.

3) d.

Post-operative intestinal obstruction can happen anytime after a laparotomy. In this case, it is probably due to adhesions. The treatment is initially conservative but surgery may be necessary if the obstruction does not resolve or the patient develops peritonitis.

4) i.

Testicular torsion is caused by twisting of the spermatic cord structures. Torsion of the spermatic cord may interrupt blood flow to the testis and epididymis causing testicular infarction. It is a surgical emergency. It is often accompanied by lower abdominal discomfort and nausea. In contrary to epididymitis the pain gets worse on elevation of the testicle.

5) c.

Diverticulitis is caused by inflammation of diverticula of the large bowel. It is more common in older patients and in the sigmoid colon. Diverticula are outpuchings of the mucosa through the muscle layers. They can get inflamed and can perforate causing localised abscesses or generalised peritonitis.

EMQ 4

a. Absence of bowel sounds
b. Board-like rigidity
c. Caput medusae
d. Grey-Turner's sign
e. Guarding
f. Murphy's sign
g. Abdominal fistula
h. Rovsing's sign
i. Shifting dullness
j. "Tinkling" bowel sounds

For each of the following scenarios, select the most characteristic clinical findings:

1) A middle-aged woman, known to have gallstones, develops severe right upper abdominal pain which has been present for 24 hours. She is pyrexial.
2) One of the medical students has developed right-sided lower abdominal pain, nausea and loss of appetite two days ago. He is unwell and very tender on examination. Tapping his abdomen over MacBurney's point causes an intense pain.
3) An elderly pub owner has developed jaundice. On inspection, his abdomen is very distended and abnormal veins are visible around his umbilicus.
4) A teenager complaining of lower abdominal pain since last evening presents with abdominal tenderness. On palpation of the left iliac fossa, he strangely reports pain on the opposite side.
5) After a heavy meal and a few bottles of wine, a usually jovial, race horse owner has become gravely ill with abdominal and back pain two days ago. He has been transferred to the intensive care unit. When you examine him he has developed dark bruising of his flanks.

Answers

> **1) f.**
> This is positive in cholecystitis. Murphy, an American surgeon, found that if one puts his hand on the patient's abdomen, below the inferior liver edge and the examined takes a deep breath in, it causes an acute pain as the inflamed gallbladder descends onto the examining hand.

2) e.

Guarding is involuntary contraction of the abdominal muscles overlying an inflamed organ or peritonitis. Guarding and rebound tenderness are characteristic clinical findings in acute appendicitis. To test for rebound the patient can be asked to cough or the abdomen can be percussed. Palpation of the tender area followed by sudden withdrawal of the hand is a more traditional way of testing for rebound tenderness (this is why it is called rebound), but is less pleasant for the patient.

3) c.

The caput medusae is the Latin description for enlarged veins arising from around the umbilicus in patients with portal hypertension. Medusa was a figure from Greek mythology and had hair made from living snakes. Caput means head in Latin.

4) h.

In 1907 N. T. Rovsing, a Danish surgeon, described that pressure on the descending and sigmoid colon in the left iliac fossa causes pain in MacBurney's point (one-third down on the line between the umbilicus and superior anterior iliac spine) — the landmark for the appendix in the right iliac fossa.

5) d.

Grey Turner, a surgeon from Newcastle-upon-Tyne, described a subcutaneous haemorrhage into the flanks in patients with haemorrhagic pancreatitis, causing local discolouration of the skin of the loins.

EMQ 5

a. ERCP
b. Hartman's resection
c. Insertion of Senkstaken tube
d. Laparoscopy
e. Midline incision
f. Partial gastrectomy
g. Repair of abdominal aneurysm
h. Right subcostal incision
i. Splenectomy
j. Small bowel resection

For each of the following patients choose the most appropriate surgical procedure:

1) A 70-year-old obese man is found by his wife collapsed on the floor. By the time they arrive at the hospital, he has improved but looks very pale and is confused. When you examine his abdomen, he denies having pain but is tender over a mass in his upper abdomen. His wife tells you that he has been complaining of back pain the whole afternoon. His blood pressure is 80 mmHg systolic.

2) A 78-year-old woman presents unwell with lower abdominal pain initially which later becomes generalised. Her abdomen is diffusely tender and you can feel some fullness in her left iliac fossa. She has a history of diverticular disease.

3) An elderly woman presents with jaundice, fever, rigours and abdominal pain.

4) A 35-year-old housewife with longstanding upper abdominal pains and known gallstones wants to be treated. She prefers open surgery.

5) A pedestrian, who has been hit by a pushbike and fallen onto the ground, presents with left-sided bruising over his lower ribs. By the time you arrive at the hospital he has become hypotensive and the ultrasound scan shows that his spleen is fragmented.

Answers

1) g.
Any elderly patient with sudden onset of back or abdominal pain and hypotension has a leaking AAA unless proven otherwise. Always have high index of suspicion because the classic presentation of pain associated with hypotension, tachycardia, and a pulsatile abdominal mass is not always present. Patients in shock are sometimes confused and denial of pain should not reassure you.

2) b.
Initially localised but then generalised abdominal pain and tenderness is typical for a localised inflammatory process causing diffuse peritonitis. A laparotomy is nearly always required. Hartmann was a French surgeon, who described the resection of a rectal carcinoma with oversewing of the rectal stump and end colostomy in 1923. This is often a safer procedure than a primary anastomosis when there is faecal contamination of the peritoneum. The lower large bowel does not heal well in the presence of sepsis.

3) a.

Jaundice, rigours and abdominal pain are a triad described in 1877 by Charcot in relation to cholangitis. The infection of the bile is usually due to a stone in the bile duct, causing biliary obstruction. Rigours are due to involuntary muscle contractions in an attempt of the body to raise the temperature to combat infection.

4) h.

The treatment for symptomatic gallstones is a cholecystectomy. The removal of the stones is not enough since the gallbladder will form new ones. Laparoscopic cholecystectomy has now replaced open cholecystectomy in the majority of cases. Open cholecystectomy may still be indicated in difficult cases or when laparoscopic chole-cystectomy has been attempted and has failed or in this case when the patient expresses a wish. The first laparoscopic cholecystectomy was performed in 1987 by Phillipe Mouret (a gynaecologist!) in France and the procedure has since become accepted as the mainstay treatment of uncomplicated gallstone disease. The traditional incision is the right subcostal described first in 1892 by Kocher, a Swiss surgeon.

5) i.

A laparotomy in an unstable patient with a ruptured spleen is a life-saving procedure. Partial conservation of the spleen in a young patient may well be an option.

Chapter 6   Breast Surgery

Rehan Saif, Muhammad Ahmed and Tom Lennard

Multiple Choice Questions

[Each single best answer (SBA) question comprises a stem and a number of answers. You are asked to decide which single item represents the best answer to the question.]

1. **The female breast**

    a) Is a modified sweat gland
    b) Is deep to the pectoral fascia
    c) Consists of 30–40 lobules
    d) The nipples contain sweat glands
    e) The axillary tail is an abnormal condition of the breast

[Best Answer = a]

Explanation

> The breast consists of 15–20 lobules. Two-thirds of the breast rests on, and hence is superficial to the deep pectoral fascia, the other third rests on the fascia covering the serratus anterior. Its lower medial edge may overlap the upper part of the rectus sheath. The skin of the breast is connected to the underlying pectoral fascia by fibrous bands called ligaments of Cooper. Their involvement in malignant process leads to skin tethering. The lobules drain by lactiferous ducts onto the nipple. The nipples are devoid of fat, hair and sweat glands. A small part of the breast may extend along the inferolateral edge of the pectoralis major towards the axilla to form the axillary tail. This may be well developed and mistaken for a breast lump or enlarged lymph nodes.

2. **The female breast**

    a) Derives its arterial supply from the internal thoracic artery only
    b) Lymphatic drainage is to the axillary lymph nodes and lymph nodes along the internal thoracic vessels
    c) The axilla contains five to ten lymph nodes

d) The pectoralis major divides the axillary lymph nodes into three levels
e) The sentinel lymph node is the last lymph node draining the tumour bearing area of the breast

[Best Answer = b]

Explanation

The breast receives its arterial supply through branches of the internal thoracic artery (anterior intercostal branches), axillary artery (lateral thoracic and thoracoacromial arteries) and intercostal arteries (lateral perforating branches). Generally, there is a tendency for the lateral part of the breast to drain to the axillary nodes, and the medial part to the nodes along the internal thoracic artery. There are connections between the two groups within the same and the contralateral breast. There are approximately 20–30 lymph nodes in the axilla, which receive approximately 85% of the drainage. They are arranged in five groups: lateral — along the axillary vein; anterior — along the lateral thoracic vessels; posterior — along the subscapular vessels; central — embedded in the axillary fat; and apical — above pectoralis minor, and into which the other nodes drain. The pectoralis minor divides the axillary lymph nodes into Level I (inferior to the muscle), Level II (behind the muscle) and Level III (above the muscle). The sentinel node is the first lymph node draining the tumour bearing area of the breast.

3. **With regards to the breast**

   a) Pre-pubertal breast structure differs between the sexes
   b) Mastitis of infants occurs only in female babies
   c) Thelarche is the beginning of breast development at puberty
   d) Under normal circumstances, both the female breasts are always symmetrical
   e) The adrenal gland controls breast development at puberty

[Best Answer = c]

Explanation

> The pre-pubertal breast is identical in both sexes and consists of a number of small ducts embedded in a collagenous stroma. The ducts develop *in utero* from an ectodermal mammary ridge. Mastitis of infants is common in both males and females. A colourless to a slightly milky secretion may be expressed from the breast in the first week of life. Also known as "witch's milk", it is considered to be due to stimulation of the foetal breast by maternal prolactin. The onset of breast development in a female starts at an average age of 10.5 years, and follows a well-ordered sequence as described by Marshall and Tanner. Hormones from the ovaries, adrenals and pituitary are important. Considerable asymmetry is frequently found among normal women, although they may not be aware of it. One-half of women may have a volume difference of 10% between the two breasts, with the left being larger in most cases.

4. **Breast screening**

    a) Is routinely offered to women between the ages 40–60 years
    b) Has been shown to reduce mortality from breast cancer
    c) Involves taking a single radiograph of the breast
    d) A screening test is generally useful for rare diseases in the population
    e) Has no morbidity

[Best Answer = b]

Explanation

> At present, screening is offered to women between 50 and 70 years (previously up to 64 years). Routine screening is not offered to women under 50. Interpretation of a mammogram in pre-menopausal women (average 50 years in UK) is difficult due to increased density of the breasts. Moreover, breast cancer is far more common in the over 50s, and the reduction in mortality with breast screening is greatest in women aged 50–70 (29%). Hence these are the targets in the screening programme. It is estimated that 1400 lives in the UK are being

saved each year due to screening. Two views of the breast are taken, craniocaudal and mediolateral. Two mammographic views have demonstrated a 42% increase in the detection of small carcinomas compared to a single view. For a screening test to be useful, the disease should be fairly common in the population, the screening test should be simple, cheap, reliable and identify those with disease and exclude those without disease. Morbidity includes the induction of anxiety in the women and a small number of negative biopsies as well as a small radiation exposure.

5. **Regarding investigations of the breast**

   a) Triple assessment is a reliable test for diagnosing breast cancer
   b) Mammographic interpretation is easier in young women
   c) Mammography involves the exposure to a high radiation dose
   d) Fine needle aspiration cytology (FNAC) is always reliable
   e) Ultrasound is an effective screening tool

[Best Answer = a]

Explanation

Triple assessment consists of a combination of clinical assessment, radiological imaging and tissue sampling for cytological or histological analysis. The positive predictive value of this assessment for cancer should exceed 99.9%, and is offered, where available, as a one-stop clinic. Mammography involves a very low radiation dose (0.1 cGy) and is considered safe. The mammographic features of a carcinoma include asymmetry, true microcalcification and stellate configuration. FNAC has a false positive rate of about two per thousand. It is dependent on both the operator and the cytologist. Moreover, it cannot differentiate invasive cancer from *in situ* disease. Ultrasound is useful particularly in the assessment of young women with dense breasts, and in distinguishing cysts from solid lesions. It is however a totally unproven screening tool.

6. Breast abscesses

a) Occur only in lactating women
b) The common causative organism is Streptococcus
c) A breast abscess must always be incised
d) May indicate an underlying carcinoma
e) Requires breast-feeding to stop

[Best Answer = d]

Explanation

Breast abscesses may occur in both lactating and non-lactating women. *Staphylococcus aureus* is the most common organism isolated. Treatment involves the use of antibiotics in the cellulitic stage. Continuation of breast-feeding is recommended if lactating, although this is controversial. Routine incision is no longer recommended for abscesses. The current recommendation is for the abscess to be aspirated repeatedly under antibiotic cover, although in persistent collections incision and drainage remains the treatment of choice.

7. Peri-ductal mastitis

a) Is less common in smokers
b) May give rise to abscess and fistula
c) Is associated with carcinoma
d) Often the discharge is milky
e) Antibiotics definitively cure the condition

[Best Answer = b]

Explanation

The pathogenesis of this condition is obscure, although cigarette smoking has been implicated. One or more of the larger lactiferous ducts may be dilated and filled with a brownish/green discharge and sometimes the condition mimics cancer. Nipple discharge is common and sometimes there is a slit-like nipple retraction. A mammary duct fistula is the development of a communication between the skin and a breast duct and is a common chronic complication of peri-ductal mastitis. Complete excision of the fistula with its associated duct is the treatment of choice.

8. **Which of the following is not involved in the treatment of cyclical mastalgia?**

    a) Exclude cancer and reassure
    b) Use of a supportive bra
    c) Oil of evening primrose
    d) Bromocriptine
    e) Surgical excision

[Best Answer = e]

Explanation

Mastalgia may be cyclical (second or third) or non-cyclical (first or third — unrelated to menstrual cycle). Cyclical pain is often bilateral, usually most severe in the upper outer quadrants of the breast, and may be referred to the medial aspect of the upper arm. Non-cyclical pain may be caused by true breast pain or chest wall pain located over the costal cartilages. Up to 70% of women develop breast pain in their lifetime. Overall, 92% of patients with cyclical mastalgia and 64% with non-cyclical mastalgia can obtain relief of their pain with therapy, though many popular remedies are of unproven benefit in randomised clinical trials.

9. **Retraction of nipple**

    a) Does not cause problems with breast feeding
    b) A long-standing slit-like retraction is characteristic of benign disease
    c) Is not seen in inflammatory breast conditions
    d) Always indicates an underlying carcinoma
    e) Can be a congenital condition

[Best Answer = b]

Explanation

Retraction of nipple may occur at puberty or later in life. In about 25%, it is bilateral and may cause problems with breast-feeding and infection can occur during lactation. It occurs in association with breast cancer and inflammatory conditions like duct ectasia and periductal mastitis. A slit-like retraction of the nipple is characteristic of benign disease and long-standing retraction has no sinister significance. A retraction that has developed recently must be regarded to be due to a cancer until proven otherwise. All patients should have a full clinical examination and if over 35 a mammogram. Duct excision can be successful at everting the nipple if it is unsightly and fails to respond to conservative measures, though subsequent scarring behind the nipple can cause inversion to recur.

10. Clinical examination of the breast

    a)   The most common sign and symptom of breast disease is a palpable mass
    b)   Clinical assessment of axillary nodes is very accurate
    c)   A bloody nipple discharge rules out malignancy
    d)   Ulceration of the skin is an early finding in breast cancer
    e)   Examination of the abdomen is an accurate method for picking up metastases

[Best Answer = a]

Explanation

Palpable axillary nodes can be identified in up to 30% of patients with no clinically significant breast or other disease, and up to 40% of patients with breast cancer who have clinically normal axillary nodes actually have axillary nodal metastases. A bloody nipple discharge can be a sign of malignancy but is usually a sign of benign intraductal papilloma. Fixation of mass to skin or chest wall and ulceration of the skin are late findings of breast cancer along with supraclavicular lymphadenopathy, oedema of the arm; bone, lung, liver, brain and other distant metastases. Examination is however a poor method for diagnosing metastases. Breast examination should include inspection in good light with the arms by the side, above the head and pressing on the hips as skin dimpling or a change in contour in the lower part of the breast is only evident when the arms are elevated or pectoral muscles are contracted.

11. Breast cancer

a) The incidence rate has fallen in the last ten years in the UK
b) Is the most common cancer in females in England
c) Is the most common cause of breast problems in patients attending breast clinics
d) Is not seen in women less than 25 years of age
e) Incidence is lowest in the developed world

[Best Answer = b]

Explanation

One in nine women will develop breast cancer at some point in their lives. The peak incidence is in the 50–64 age group. It is also the most common cause of cancer death in women and the incidence is highest in the developed world. Interestingly migrants from low to high risk countries acquire the risk of the host country within two generations. With the introduction of breast screening programme in 1988, the incidence of breast cancer has actually increased, probably because cancers are being picked up earlier than they were before screening was introduced. It is extremely rare below the age of 25, but thereafter the incidence rises with age. Benign breast disease is the most common cause of breast problems — up to 30% of women will suffer from a benign breast disorder requiring treatment at some time in their lives.

12. Risk factors in breast cancer

a) It is more common in multiparous women
b) Having a first child at an early age is protective
c) Previous benign breast disease is not a risk factor

d) Up to 40% of breast cancer is due to genetic predisposition
e) Not related to diet and lifestyle

[Best Answer = b]

Explanation

Nulliparity and late age at first pregnancy both increase the lifetime incidence of breast cancer. The risk is doubled in women who have their first child after the age of 30. Women with atypical epithelial hyperplasia have four to five times higher risk of developing breast cancer than women who do not have any proliferative changes in their breast. A woman's risk of breast cancer is two or more times greater if she has a first degree relative (mother, sister or daughter) who developed the disease before the age of 50. Up to 10% of breast cancer is due to genetic predisposition. There is some evidence that breast cancer is related to a high intake of alcohol, increased fat intake and obesity. This is thought to be because of increased conversion of steroid hormones to oestradiol in body fat.

13. Pathology of breast cancer

a) Breast cancer arises in the proximal duct lobular unit
b) Lobular carcinoma is the least common variant
c) Inflammatory breast cancer carries a better prognosis
d) Medullary cancer carries a worse prognosis
e) Invasive lobular carcinoma is the most common type to be bilateral

[Best Answer = e]

Explanation

Breast cancers are derived from the epithelial cells that line the terminal duct lobular unit. It may be entirely *in situ* — pre-invasive cancer (increasingly detected with screening) or may be invasive cancer. Inflammatory breast cancer is a fortunately rare, highly aggressive cancer which presents as a painful, swollen breast and may mimic a breast abscess. Rarer histological variants like medullary carcinoma, colloid carcinoma and tubular carcinoma usually carry a better prognosis. Lobular carcinoma occurs in up to 10% of cases, the most common variant being ductal carcinoma.

14. Clinical presentation of carcinoma of the breast

a) It commences most frequently in the inner lower quadrant
b) Peau d'orange is a sign of early disease
c) Most common presentation is a painful lump
d) All patients should have a tissue diagnosis prior to definitive surgery
e) Treatment does not depend on axillary node status

[Best Answer = d]

Explanation

Sixty per cent of all breast lumps commence in the upper outer quadrant. Peau d'orange is due to cutaneous lymphatic oedema giving the appearance of an orange skin and is a sign of advanced disease. Most breast cancers will present as a painless hard lump. Axillary node status remains the single best prognostic factor and important treatment decisions are based upon it.

15. Breast reconstruction

a) Reconstruction makes diagnosis of recurrent cancer difficult
b) Immediate reconstruction increases the psychological trauma after mastectomy
c) Use of a silicone gel implant under the pectoralis major muscle is the most common type of reconstruction
d) Infection rarely occurs after latissimus dorsi flaps
e) Flap necrosis occurs in 40% of myocutaneous flap reconstructions

[Best Answer = c]

Explanation

Reconstruction is not an obstacle to the diagnosis of recurrent cancer. It should probably be discussed with patients prior to mastectomy, because it offers an important psychological focal point for recovery. The options for breast reconstruction are prosthesis, tissue expansion along with prosthesis and myocutaneous flaps. The two most common myocutaneous flaps used require movement of either the latissimus dorsi muscle with overlying skin or the lower abdominal fat and skin based on the rectus abdominis muscle [transverse rectus abdominis myocutaneous (TRAM) flap]. Flap necrosis occurs in up to 10% of patients with TRAM flaps but is rare after a latissimus dorsi myocutaneous flap where infection is more of a problem. Removal of the rectus abdominis causes abdominal hernias in about 5% of patients. Implants can be saline or silicone filled. There has been controversy about the risks of abnormal immune responses with silicone, although in the UK silicone is still the most popular implant because of its natural consistency (compared with saline) and nowadays all implants used in the UK are on a form which is sent to the UK Breast Implant Registry.

Case Studies

Case 1

A 22-year-old male presents with a bilateral painless enlargement of the breasts. On examination, both his breasts appear to be enlarged with prominent infra-mammary folds.

a) What is the likely diagnosis?
b) What are the causes for this condition in general?
c) How will you investigate this patient?
d) What medical treatment can you offer?
e) Is surgical treatment an option in this condition?

Answers

a) The most likely diagnosis is gynaecomastia.
b) Gynaecomastia can be idiopathic, physiologic or pathologic. Physiologic gynaecomastia may be seen in newborn infants, pubertal adolescents, and elderly individuals. Pathologic gynae-comastia may be caused by a decreased production or action of testosterone (Klinefelters syndrome, renal failure, androgen insensitivity) or to increased production or action of estrogens (testicular tumour, chronic liver disease). Drugs such as cimetidine, digoxin and spironolactone have also been implicated.
c) A thorough history and physical examination may reveal the underlying cause. Physiological gynaecomastia often requires no further investigation. Depending on the clinical situation, the following blood tests may be requested: serum chemistry for chronic liver and renal diseases, tests for thyroid function, and levels of gonadal hormones. Imaging requested may include mammography and testicular ultrasound. Fine needle aspiration cytology or biopsy may be required.
d) Reassurance may be all that is required in adolescent cases. When caused by drugs, withdrawal or change of the drug should be considered.
e) Subcutaneous mastectomy may be offered to the patients. This involves preservation of the nipple and areola.

Case 2

A 38-year-old woman presents with bilateral breast pain, worse before her periods. She regularly performs self-examination of the breast and has not noticed any lump.

a) What is the most likely diagnosis?
b) What are its causes?
c) What is the difference between cyclical and non-cyclical mastalgia?
d) What is the treatment for the condition?

Answers

a) The most likely diagnosis is cyclical mastalgia.
b) It is thought that women with cyclical breast pain have breast tissue, which is more sensitive than usual to the normal hormonal changes, which occur each month. It is not considered to be due to any hormonal disease, or to any problem in the breast itself.
c) Mastalgia may be cyclical (second or third) or non-cyclical (first or third — unrelated to menstrual cycle). Cyclical pain is often bilateral, usually most severe in the upper outer quadrants of the breast, and may be referred to the medial aspect of the upper arm. It tends to develop from about mid-cycle onwards, and is usually worse for three to seven days before a period. The severity can vary from month to month. Quality of life for some women can be quite affected. Physical activity such as jogging, hugging children and sexual activity may be painful. Non-cyclical pain may be caused by true breast pain or chest wall pain located over the costal cartilages.
e) Reassurance that cancer is not responsible for the symptoms helps a lot of patients. The use of a well-supported bra is encouraged. There is some anecdotal evidence that reducing caffeine intake may help. The drugs that are licensed for use in cyclical mastalgia include danazol and bromocriptine. Tamoxifen is also effective in treating cyclical mastalgia, though it is not licensed for use in this condition in the UK.

Case 3

A 55-year-old lady presented with a painless lump in her right breast with no fixity to the skin. Mammography and cytology confirmed this to be malignant. She was scheduled for surgery, and she chose a wide local excision to be performed along with sentinel node biopsy.

a) What is a sentinel lymph node?
b) What is its significance in breast cancer?
c) How is sentinel lymph node biopsy performed?
d) Why is sentinel lymph node biopsy performed?
e) What happens if the sentinel lymph node is found to be cancerous?

Answers

a) The "sentinel" node is the very first lymph node(s) to receive drainage from a cancer-containing area of the breast.
b) Preliminary studies suggest that if no cancer cells are found in the sentinel node, the patient is unlikely to have tumour cells in the remaining axillary nodes.
c) There are two methods for finding the sentinel node. One is to inject a blue dye near the breast tumour and track its path through the lymph nodes. The dye accumulates in the sentinel node. In a similar technique, a small amount of a radioactive solution is injected near the tumour and a gamma detector is used to find the "hotspot", or the node in which the solution has accumulated. These two techniques can also be used together to optimise localisation.
d) Standard treatment for breast cancer usually involves removing the breast tumor by either wide excision or mastectomy and removing most of the axillary nodes (axillary node dissection) to stage the cancer. Axillary node dissection is associated with increased morbidity. Studies suggest that if an analysis finds no cancer cells in the sentinel node, the patient is unlikely to have tumour cells in the remaining axillary nodes. Most patients have only one to three sentinel lymph nodes under the arm. Thus, an average of only two lymph nodes is removed in each patient with a sentinel node biopsy. This, in turn, may reduce post-operative complications.
e) If the sentinel lymph node is found to be cancerous, then additional surgery may be necessary to remove more nodes for examination.

Case 4

A 54-year-old woman presents with a lump in her right breast in the upper outer quadrant.

a) What is the most likely diagnosis and how should the patient be managed initially?
b) What investigations should be performed?
c) What are the principles of management?
d) What are the risk factors for development of metastatic disease?
e) What are the complications of surgery?

Answers

a) The most likely diagnosis is carcinoma of breast. A good history and full clinical examination should be carried out. Doing an FNAC and mammogram should complete triple assessment. Once the diagnosis is made, the extent of disease should be assessed and the tumour staged according to the UICC classification (TNM).

b) To ensure that there is no gross evidence of disease, all patients should have a full blood count, liver function tests and a chest radiograph. Patients with stage I and II disease ($T_1N_0M_0$, $T_1N_1M_0$, $T_2N_{0-1}M_0$) have a low incidence of detectable metastatic disease and in the absence of abnormal LFTs need not undergo further investigations. Patients with bigger or more advanced tumours should be considered for bone and liver scans if these could lead to a change in clinical management.

c) Most patients will have a combination of local treatments to control local disease and systemic treatment for any micrometastatic disease. Tumours less than 4 cm are suitable for breast conserving surgery. It consists of excision of the tumour with a 1 cm margin or normal tissue (wide local excision) or a more extensive excision of a whole quadrant of the breast (quadrantectomy). Patients undergoing breast conservation surgery should receive radiotherapy to the remaining breast tissue. For bigger tumours (in relation to size of the breast), central tumours beneath or involving the nipple, multifocal disease, local recurrence or patient preference, a simple mastectomy is done. Mastectomy should be combined with some form of axillary surgery to stage the axilla, as the presence of metastatic disease within the axillary lymph nodes is still the best marker for prognosis. Adjuvant systemic therapy in the form of hormonal therapy or chemotherapy has been shown to improve survival. Choice of treatment depends on risk of relapse, potential benefits of different treatments, oestrogen receptor status and acceptability of treatment to the patient. Age or menopausal status is the other important factor that affects the choice of adjuvant treatment. Tamoxifen is the most widely used hormonal therapy and its effect is favourable in most cases except for oestrogen-receptor negative (ER-negative) women. Optimal duration of treatment is five years. Other hormonal agents have been developed such as the aromatase inhibitors and LHRH agonists. The benefits of chemotherapy are greater in women aged under 50 than in older women. Adjuvant chemotherapy is now widely used in women over the age of 50 but is rarely given to women over the age of 70.

d) The major risk factors for development of subsequent metastatic disease are presence of involved axillary lymph nodes, a poor histological grade (indicating an undifferentiated cancer) and large tumour size.

e) Complications after mastectomy include formation of seroma, infection and flap necrosis. Complications following axillary surgery include damage to nerves, most commonly the intercostobrachial nerve causing numbness and paraesthesiae down the upper inner aspect of the arm, wound infection and lymphoedema.

Case 5

A 60-year-old woman presents to the clinic with eczematoid change of the left nipple and areola. She received a topical steroid application from her GP but the condition persisted and the nipple eventually eroded.

a) What is the most likely diagnosis?
b) What condition does it mimic and how can it be differentiated?
c) What investigations should be done?
d) How would you manage this condition?

Answers

a) The most likely diagnosis is Paget's disease of the nipple. It is a superficial manifestation of an underlying carcinoma.

b) It mimics eczema of the nipple. Eczema is bilateral and usually affects the areolar region first and only rarely affects the nipple skin. It responds to local topical treatment. Paget's disease affects the nipple from the start.

c) A good history and full clinical examination should be carried out. In half of these patients, it is associated with an underlying mass lesion. Mammography should be performed to determine if there is an underlying lesion. Imprint cytology or scrape cytology can sometimes establish the diagnosis. The most reliable method of obtaining a diagnosis is by incisional biopsy.

d) If a mass lesion is present and remote from the nipple, the appropriate treatment is mastectomy and axillary node clearance. When Paget's disease is associated with an underlying central lesion, a wide excision of the nipple, areola and underlying mass followed by radiotherapy can give a reasonable cosmetic result and satisfactory control of local disease. For patients without a mass lesion, wide local excision followed by radiotherapy produces satisfactory local control rates.

Extended Matching Questions

EMQ 1

a. Duct papilloma
b. Mondor's disease
c. Traumatic fat necrosis
d. Fibroadenoma
e. Amazia
f. Diffuse hypertrophy
g. Breast cyst
h. Fibroadenosis
i. Milk fistula
j. Gynaecomastia
k. Breast abscess

Choose the diagnosis from the list above, which most fits the case scenarios described below:

1) A woman presents with a sudden appearance of a linear, cordlike, fibrous band under the left breast.
2) A 16-year-old male presents with a bilateral enlargement of the breast.
3) A 45-year-old woman presents with a discrete lump. Fine needle aspiration yields a clear fluid and a complete resolution of the lump.
4) An 18-year-old girl presents with a discreet, mobile lump in her right breast.
5) A 45-year-old woman presents with generalised lumpiness in the upper outer quadrants of both her breasts. She also describes pain that is worse pre-menstrually.
6) A 32-year-old lactating woman presents with a three-day history of an erythematous, tender area in her right breast.

Answers

> **1) b.**
> Mondor's disease is characterised by the sudden appearance of a subcutaneous cord, which is initially red and tender and subsequently becomes a painless, tough, fibrous band. The cord is accentuated by traction, elevation of the breast, or abduction of the ipsilateral arm. The condition, though benign and self-limited, has been rarely associated with breast cancer.

2) j.

Gynaecomastia is the growth of the male breast tissue to any extent in all ages. It is usually reversible and benign. Reassurance and removal of the cause, e.g. drugs, may be sufficient.

3) g.

Breast cysts are often firm, smooth and fairly discrete (15% of all discrete breast masses). They do not require any further treatment if, on aspiration, it resolves completely and the aspirate is not blood stained; 1%–3% of breast cysts have carcinomas. Any residual mass after aspiration requires further assessment.

4) d.

Fibroadenomas are the most common benign tumours of the female breast. They develop at any age but are more common in young women. They account for approximately 13% of all palpable symptomatic breast masses. They do not require excision routinely as less than 10% of them will grow over a two-year period.

5) h.

Fibroadenosis or fibrocystic disease is the most common cause of breast lumps in women of reproductive age. The peak incidence is between 35 and 50 years of age. It usually presents with a single lump or *features* multiple lumps in the upper outer quadrant of the breast that are painful and tender premenstrually (i.e. cyclical). Provided that imaging (ultrasound or mammography) and FNAC have eliminated a malignancy, essentially the treatment is reassurance and medication for symptom relief.

6) k.

Breast abscesses may occur in both lactating and non-lactating women. *Staphylococcus aureus* is the most common organism isolated. Treatment involves the use of antibiotics in the cellulitic stage. Continuation of breast feeding is recommended if lactating, although this is controversial. Routine incision is no longer recommended for abscesses. The current recommendation is for the abscess to be aspirated repeatedly under antibiotic cover.

EMQ 2

a. Mammography and cytology
b. Ultrasound
c. Fine needle aspiration cytology
d. Cytology of discharge
e. Occult blood test
f. Core biopsy
g. Excision biopsy
h. Repeated aspiration
i. Incision and drainage
j. Subcutaneous mastectomy
k. Reassurance

Select the most appropriate initial investigation(s) or treatment option(s) for the patients described below:

1) A young woman presents with a two-day history of an indurated, tender area in her left breast. There is no history of trauma.
2) A 23-year-old girl presents with a well-defined mobile lump in her left breast. She noticed this four months ago and has not noticed any change in its size with her cycles.
3) A 45-year-old woman presents with a discrete lump. Fine needle aspiration yields a clear fluid and a complete resolution of the lump.
4) A 40-year-old lady presents with a hard lump in her right breast. She describes sustaining an injury to her breast recently.

Answers

> **1) b.**
> Ultrasound. This is likely to be developing breast abscess. In the early cellulitic phase, antibiotics may lead to a complete resolution. Once pus formation has occurred, repeated aspiration with antibiotic cover will be required. Ultrasound can be useful in demonstrating pus if this is not obvious clinically and allow any pus to be drained using image guidance. Incision and drainage under general anaesthesia may be required if resolution does not occur.
>
> **2) b.**
> Ultrasound. This is a better investigative tool in young women with dense breast than mammography. Fibroadenomas may be left alone if

cytology and ultrasound confirm that they are benign. Excision biopsy may be undertaken if they are large (>4 cm), of suspicious cytology, occur in women over 40 years or due to patient's wishes.

3) k.
Reassurance only. This is a benign breast cyst. If the cyst aspirate is clear and the cyst regresses completely, no further investigation or treatment is required other than reassurance that this is a simple breast cyst. If there is a residual lump on re-examination after the aspiration, full assessment with mammography and fine needle aspiration cytology would then be indicated.

4) a.
Fat necrosis may mimic a carcinoma with the presence of a hard lump and skin tethering. Diagnosis requires a triple assessment — history and examination, mammography and fine needle aspiration cytology. Excision biopsy may be required in some cases to exclude malignancy with certainty.

EMQ 3

a. Peau d'orange
b. Ductal carcinoma *in situ* (DCIS)
c. Duct ectasia
d. Phyllodes tumour
e. Metastatic breast cancer
f. Inflammatory breast cancer
g. Cancer-en-cuirasse

Choose the diagnosis from the list above, which most fits the case scenarios described below:

1) A 62-year-old woman who previously underwent a mastectomy for breast cancer presents with local recurrence infiltrating the skin of the chest.
2) A 57-year-old lady presents with a lump in her left breast. On examination, the skin over the lump gives the appearance of an orange skin.
3) A 55-year-old lady presents with a painful, swollen right breast which is warm with cutaneous oedema.
4) A 70-year-old lady who previously underwent a mastectomy for breast cancer presents with a fracture of the right femur following a trivial fall.

5) A 60-year-old woman underwent a screening mammogram which revealed microcalcification.

Answers

1) g.
This usually occurs in cases with local recurrence after mastectomy. It may be associated with a grossly swollen arm. The skin of the chest is infiltrated with carcinoma and has been likened to a coat. It may respond to palliative systemic treatment or radiotherapy but prognosis in terms of survival is poor.

2) a.
Peau d'orange is due to cutaneous lymphatic oedema. Where the infiltrated skin is tethered it cannot swell, leading to the appearance like orange skin. It is a sign of advanced breast cancer. Occasionally the same phenomenon is seen over a chronic abscess.

3) f.
Inflammatory breast cancer is a fortunately rare, highly aggressive cancer, which presents as a painful, swollen breast, which is warm with cutaneous oedema. This is due to blockage of subdermal lymphatics with carcinoma cells. It may mimic a breast abscess. A biopsy will confirm the diagnosis.

4) e.
Mammary carcinoma spreads by local spread, lymphatic spread and spread by the bloodstream. It is by the haematogenous route that skeletal metastases occur (in order of frequency) in the lumbar vertebrae, femur, thoracic vertebrae, rib and skull. Metastases may also occur in the liver, lung and brain, and occasionally the adrenal glands and ovaries.

5) b.
Screen detected carcinoma is most commonly associated with microcalcification, which is characteristic of DCIS.

EMQ 4

a. Galactocele
b. Phyllodes tumour
c. Amazia
d. Polymazia
e. Diffuse hypertrophy
f. Duct papilloma
g. Fibroadenoma
h. Breast cysts
i. Gynaecomastia
j. Diffuse hypertrophy of the breast

Choose the diagnosis from the list above, which most fits the case scenarios described below:

1) Congenital absence of the breast.
2) Treated by reduction mammoplasty.
3) Treated by microdochectomy or cone excision.
4) A retention cyst that results from occlusion of a lactiferous duct.
5) Usually benign but may recur locally.

Answers

1) c.
Congenital absence of the breast may occur on one or both sides. When associated with absence of the sternal portion of pectoralis major, it is termed Poland's syndrome.

2) e.
Diffuse hypertrophy of the breasts occurs at puberty or during the first pregnancy in otherwise healthy girls.

3) f.
Duct papilloma may be single or multiple. They are very common and often present with nipple discharge, which is often blood stained. Simple assurance may be sufficient once a carcinoma has been excluded. Surgical treatment may be offered if discharge is intolerable, and is often needed to exclude carcinoma.

EMQ 5

a. Follicle stimulating hormone
b. Prolactin
c. Oxytocin
d. Estrogen
e. Luteinising hormone
f. Relaxin
g. Thyroid stimulation hormone
h. Progesterone

Choose the hormone from the list above which best describes its effects below:

1) Mainly responsible for the enlargement of the female breast at puberty.
2) Causes development of the lobule and alveoli.
3) Responsible for the milk ejection reflex.
4) Regulates milk secretion.

Answers

1) d.
Estrogens produce duct growth in the breasts and are largely responsible for breast enlargement at puberty in girls.

2) h.
Progesterone stimulates the development of lobules and alveoli. It induces the differentiation of estrogen-prepared ductal tissue and supports the secretory function of the breast during lactation.

3) c.
Oxytocin causes contraction of the myoepithelial cells lining the duct walls, with consequent ejection of milk through the nipple. Oxytocin is secreted as a result of anticipatory nursing or by sensory stimuli from the nipple-areola complex and is inhibited by pain and embarrassment.

4) b.
Prolactin is a critical factor in all phases of breast development and lactation. It synergises with progesterone in stimulating lobuloalveolar development. It regulates milk secretion, including the synthesis of milk proteins. Suckling maintains and augments the secretion of milk because of the stimulation of prolactin secretion by suckling.

Chapter 7   Head, Neck and Skin

Monica Hansrani and Nigel Jones

Multiple Choice Questions

[Each single best answer (SBA) question comprises a stem and a number of answers. You are asked to decide which single item represents the best answer to the question.]

1. **Which of the following is not found in the anterior triangle of the neck?**

    a) Thyroglossal cyst
    b) Carotid body tumour
    c) Submandibular gland
    d) Supraclavicular (Virchow's) lymph node
    e) Jugulodigastric node

[Best Answer = d]

Explanation

> The anterior triangle is bounded by the lower border of the mandible, the anterior border of the sternocleidomastoid muscle and the midline. Therefore only the carotid body tumour (chemodectoma), submandibular gland, jugulodigastric node and thyroglossal cyst lie within these boundaries, but not the supraclavicular node, which lies in the posterior triangle.

2. **In thyroid cancers**

    a) Anaplastic tumours have a good prognosis
    b) Papillary cancers present in young adults
    c) Thyroid suppression can be used to treat medullary carcinomas
    d) Lymphoma frequently develops after Hashimoto's thyroiditis
    e) Chemotherapy is the mainstay of treatment for all thyroid cancers

[Best Answer = b]

Explanation

> Anaplastic tumours are aggressive and have a very poor prognosis. Papillary cancers account for 85% of thyroid tumours and most commonly present in young adults. Medullary carcinoma is cancer of the calcitonin producing C-cells in the thyroid and therefore is not sensitive to TSH and thyroid suppression. Only 10% of patients with Hashimoto's thyroiditis develop lymphoma in the gland. Chemotherapy is not the mainstay of treatment for most thyroid cancers (surgery and radio-iodine are), but remains the primary modality of treatment in all lymphomas, which are a rare cause of thyroid cancer.

3. Branchial cysts

a) Are usually symptomatic at birth
b) Are lined with squamous epithelium
c) Twenty-five per cent are bilateral
d) Can arise from the proximal oesophagus
e) Commonly recur after excision

[Best Answer = b]

Explanation

> Branchial cysts are lined with squamous epithelium and arise from the pharyngeal wall (remnants of the second branchial cleft) and are bilateral in 2%–3% of cases. They usually present in young adults. Recurrence is uncommon after excision.

4. With respect to lumps presenting in childhood

a) Branchial cysts usually present symptomatically at birth
b) A cystic hygroma can cause stridor in babies
c) Dermoid cysts commonly occur at the angle of the mouth
d) Bronchogenic cysts present in the anterior triangle of the neck
e) Medullary carcinoma commonly presents in teenagers

[Best Answer = b]

Explanation

> Although branchial cysts are congenital, they rarely present in babies, more commonly in young adults, whilst cystic hygromas are often present at birth and may be so large as to obstruct labour and cause tracheal compression leading to stridor. Dermoid cysts are commonly found at the medial and lateral ends of the eyebrow, midline of the nose, sublingually and in the midline of the neck. These are sites of embryological fusion. Bronchogenic cysts are congenital anomalies of development of the bronchi and lungs and most often present as radio-opaque masses on chest X-rays. Medullary cancers of the thyroid rarely present in teenagers.

5. **When requested to examine the thyroid**
   a) Palpation of the thyroid gland is performed from behind the patient
   b) The neck should be extended during palpation
   c) Should include examination of the ears
   d) If no mass is felt in the gland there is no need to examine lymph nodes of the neck
   e) Does not require the use of a stethoscope

[Best Answer = a]

Explanation

> If the examiner asks you to examine the thyroid, the hands, face, eyes should also be examined for signs of hyperthyroidism (hot, sweaty palms, rapid pulse, anxiety, eye signs suggestive of Grave's disease) or hypothyroidism (dry skin, slow pulse, coarse hair, thickening of facial features). The examination of the gland should be performed from behind the patient with the neck flexed to relax the overlying sternocleidomastoid muscles. A clinically normal gland does not preclude cancer as the lesion may be small and deep. You should auscultate the gland to listen for a bruit even in small glands.

6. Papillary carcinoma of the thyroid

a) Arises from the calcitonin producing C-cells
b) Is not sensitive to radioactive iodine
c) Has a poor prognosis
d) Metastasises via the haematogenous route
e) Is the most common thyroid cancer

[Best Answer = e]

Explanation

Medullary carcinomas arise from the C-cells. Papillary carcinoma is the most common thyroid cancer (85%). It is slow growing, metastasises to the regional lymph nodes and has a good prognosis even in the presence of metastases. Diagnosis is confirmed by hemithyroidectomy. If the tumour is multifocal, greater than 1 cm in diameter or extending outside the thyroid capsule to invade other structures, then completion thyroidectomy, followed by radioactive iodine is performed.

7. Lymph nodes

The most appropriate initial investigation of bilateral lymph node enlargement in the neck in a young person is:

a) Monospot blood test
b) CT of thorax and abdomen
c) Surgical open biopsy
d) Skull X-ray
e) Sialogram

[Best Answer = a]

Explanation

The monospot is an agglutination test to measure the presence of IgM for Epstein-Barr virus which causes infectious mononucleosis, a common cause of cervical lymphadenopathy. A surgical biopsy is not appropriate as an initial investigation as a fine needle aspiration cytology (FNAC) or core biopsy will provide as much information without the requirement for a general anaesthetic and the complications of a surgical procedure. It would be inappropriately invasive as an initial investigation. An FNAC and CXR are essential for the exclusion of malignancy, however a skull X-ray is not useful. A sialogram is used for the assessment of salivary gland drainage and therefore not appropriate. CT of the thorax and abdomen form part of the staging assessment for lymphoma once this diagnosis has been made.

8. **One of the following anatomical statements is correct**

   a) The anterior triangle of the neck is bounded by the lower border of the mandible, the anterior border of trapezius and the clavicles
   b) The supraclavicular fossa lies in the anterior triangle
   c) The submental region lies below the inferior border of the mandible anteriorly
   d) The parotid gland lies in the posterior triangle of the neck
   e) The jugulodigastric lymph node lies deep to the sternocleidomastoid

[Best Answer = c]

Explanation

The anterior triangle is bounded by the lower border of the mandible, the anterior border of the sternocleidomastoid muscle and the midline. It contains the jugulodigastric node which lies superficially at the angle of the mandible. The posterior triangle is bounded by the anterior border of sternocleidomastoid, anterior border of trapezius and the clavicle. Therefore the supraclavicular fossa lies in the posterior triangle. The area anteroinferior to the mandible is indeed the submental region. The parotid gland does not lie in the neck.

9. **Follicular carcinoma of the thyroid gland**

   a) Can be diagnosed by an ultrasound of the neck and FNAC
   b) Causes 85% of thyroid cancers
   c) Metastases occur via the lymphatics

d) Growth is stimulated by thyroid stimulating hormone (TSH)

e) Presents in the elderly

[Best Answer = d]

Explanation

> Follicular carcinoma represents approximately 10% of thyroid cancers. FNAC cannot distinguish between follicular adenoma and carcinoma and therefore is not diagnostic. It presents in young and middle-aged adults, is slow growing and metastasises through the blood borne route to lungs, bone and liver. It is sensitive to TSH, and thyroid suppression therapy is important post-surgery.

10. Cystic hygroma

a) Is a mucus-containing cyst

b) Is found in the anterior triangle of the neck

c) Commonly presents in teenagers

d) Increases in size when the patient coughs or cries

e) Commonly recurs

[Best Answer = d]

Explanation

> A cystic hygroma is a lymph-containing cyst which results from maldevelopment and obstruction of the lymphatic system. It most commonly presents at birth or in the first two years of life, with a lump in the posterior triangle of the neck that increases in size when the baby cries or coughs. It can be treated with surgical excision or aspiration and injection of a sclerosant. It recurs in 10% of patients.

11. Parotid gland

a) Surgical excision can lead to damage to the Vth nerve

b) Should be bimanually palpated

c) Is usually enlarged with Epstein Barr virus infection

d) Is the most common salivary gland to be affected by calculi

e) Sialography involves mapping out the gland using ultrasound

[Best Answer = b]

Explanation

All parotid lumps should be bimanually palpated with a finger inside the mouth and one over the cheek to feel extent of any lumps and possibly palpate a lump in the duct. The facial (VIIth) nerve runs right through the gland separating it into a superficial and deep part and may be damaged during surgical excision. The salivary glands most commonly affected by duct stones (calculi) are the submandibular glands due to their long duct with a slightly uphill course. Sialography involves X-ray or CT of the gland using contrast to delineate the salivary ducts. Epstein Barr virus causes glandular fever and causes cervical lymph node enlargement. Mumps virus causes parotid enlargement.

12. In cancers of the larynx

a) Eighty per cent may be due to cigarette smoking

b) Leukoplakia is a benign condition

c) Most commonly is adenocarcinoma

d) In 50% of cases more than one cancers may be present at the same time

e) Mutation of p53 protects from the development of cancer

[Best Answer = a]

Explanation

A history of heavy smoking, often combined with heavy drinking, is found in about 80% of patients. Leukoplakia is a white plaque found in the oropharynx which is a pre-malignant condition. The most common cancer of the larynx is squamous cell cancer. In 10% of cases a second primary squamous cell carcinoma (SCC), known as a synchronous tumour may be present. P53 is an oncogene and therefore mutation can lead to the development of cancer.

13. Virchow's node

With which of the following, is enlargement of the left supraclavicular (Virchow's) lymph node not associated?

    a)   Breast adenocarcinoma
    b)   Gastric adenocarcinoma
    c)   Parotid pleomorphic adenoma
    d)   Ovarian serous carcinoma
    e)   Hepatocellular carcinoma

[Best Answer = c]

Explanation

> Enlargement of Virchow's node (known as Trosier's sign) may show evidence of metastatic spread of an otherwise asymptomatic cancer of the thorax or abdomen, as lymph drainage from the body enters the jugular vein via the thoracic duct at this point. A pleomorphic adenoma is a benign tumour of the salivary glands (usually the parotid gland) and therefore does not spread to lymph nodes.

14. In relation to scars

    a)   Surgical incisions should avoid Langer's lines
    b)   Melanoma occurring in a chronic leg ulcer is known as a Marjolin's ulcer
    c)   Psoriasis developing in a scar is known as Koebner's phenomenon
    d)   Keloids develop rarely in scars around the neck and upper chest
    e)   Keloid scars are best treated with surgical excision

[Best Answer = c]

Explanation

> Langer's lines are the lines in the direction of least stress in the skin. Incisions placed along these lines are more likely to heal with good scars, and therefore where possible the direction of Langer's lines should be taken into account when placing a scar. A Marjolin's ulcer

is a chronic ulcer in which squamous cell carcinoma has developed. A keloid is an area of overgrowth of a scar. Scars of the neck and chest wall, and burns are particularly prone to this phenomenon, particularly in people of Afro-Caribbean descent. Attempts at surgical excision are likely to exacerbate the situation; treatment is with silicone/steriod gel and pressure dressings.

15. Basal cell carcinomas

a) Usually presents in preschool children
b) Actinic keratoses often precede their development
c) Classically lesions are well demarcated erythematous plaques topped by silvery scales
d) Commonly presents in areas of sun-exposed skin such as the face and ears
e) Are often associated with arthropathy

[Best Answer = d]

Explanation

Psoriasis is a dermatological condition which classically presents with erythematous plaques topped by silvery scales on the *extensor* surfaces of the knees and elbows and scalp and can be associated with arthropathy. Basal cell carcinomas typically present as a raised small pearly dome-shaped nodule with visible vessels (telangiectasia) crossing them. They are found mainly on sun-exposed areas and commonly present in the elderly. Actinic keratoses are dry scaly rough-textured spots or patches that develop in sun-exposed skin which may progress to squamous cell carcinomas.

Case Studies

Case 1

A 32-year-woman presents as she has noticed that a pigmented mole on her thigh has increased in size, changed in colour in parts, is itchy and spontaneously bleeds.

a) What is the most likely diagnosis?
b) How would you confirm your diagnosis?
c) Describe one of the methods used to stage the disease?
d) What is a sentinel node biopsy and how is it performed?
e) Other than surgery, what other modalities of therapy are possible in this case?

Answers

a) Malignant melanoma.
b) Take a history and examination, looking for risk factors such as rapid growth, fair skin, sun exposure, an irregular margin, marked variation in colour, ulceration, lymphadenopathy; excision biopsy with a 1 cm margin, is the investigation of choice, but if the lesion is too big, incisional biopsy of several suspicious areas of the lesion can be performed although a false negative can occur due to sampling error.
c) The two commonly used systems are the Clark's levels and Breslow thickness Clark's levels.

Clark's levels		Breslow thickness
I	Epidermis only	<0.75 mm
II	Invades papillary dermis	<3.0 mm
III	Fills papillary dermis	>3.0 mm
IV	Invades reticular dermis	>4.0 mm
V	Subcutaneous tissue invasion	

Clinical stage is then given by:

IA <0.75 mm or Clark's level II
IB 0.75–1.5 mm or Clark's level III
IIA 1.4–4.0 mm or Clarke's level IV
IIB >4.0 mm or Clark's level V
III Lymph node mets in one regional drainage area or >5 in transit mets
IV Advanced regional metastases or distant metastases

d) The sentinel lymph node is the first lymph node to which the melanoma drains, therefore if this is negative, in theory there is no necessity to perform a block dissection of the regional nodes. The sentinel node is identified using a "vital dye" and a radioactive marker agent which are injected into the lesion and then following the colour and using lymphoscintography with a gamma camera to map out the progress to the first draining lymph nodes. A "block dissection" of the regional lymph nodes involves surgical removal of all of the regional lymph nodes draining the tumour leading to significant morbidity whilst yielding only positive evidence of spread in only 20% of patients.

e) Chemotherapy with or without hormone therapy (tamoxifen). Immunotherapy utilising antibodies targeting malignant melanoma cells which are labelled with cytotoxic agents are currently under evaluation. In general melanomas are not radiosensitive, but intraluminal BCG therapy with radiotherapy has shown some benefit.

Case 2

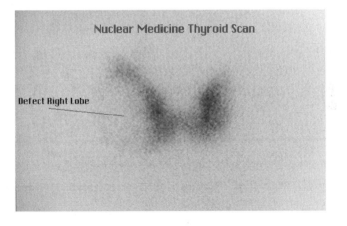

a) What does this scan show?
b) What is the differential diagnosis for this lump?
c) How else would you investigate this patient to come to the diagnosis?
d) What signs and symptoms would increase the possibility of this lesion being malignant?
e) Describe how you would consent this patient for a hemithyroidectomy? What risks would you need to consent them for?

Answers

a) The scan shows a "cold nodule", i.e. a nodule in the thyroid that does not take up the iodine-123 or technetium-99 isotope and therefore does not have functioning thyroid tissue.

b) Thyroid cyst, non-functioning adenoma, well-differentiated carcinoma, lymphoma, metastasis.

c) Take a full history and examination of the patient. Perform a fine needle aspirate cytology (FNAC) and perform an ultrasound scan of the neck.

d) The presence of lymphadenopathy, hoarseness due to recurrent laryngeal nerve palsy, persistent pain or dysphagia are suspicious signs. In addition, the younger the patient the higher the risk of malignancy and in men a thyroid lump has a much higher risk of being malignant than in a woman.

e) Ideally consent should be performed in a quiet room in the presence of a relative with adequate time allotted without disturbance. For many operations there are information sheets that can be provided. You will need to describe the operation — that it will involve a transverse incision in the lower neck, that half of the thyroid will be removed. They may have a drain placed in their neck for 24 hours. The risks quoted are of haemorrhage, potentially requiring urgent return to theatre; hoarseness or obstructive breathing (recurrent laryngeal nerve injury), a change in quality of the voice (superior laryngeal nerve injury); risk of hypocalcaemia.

Case 3

A 60-year-old man presents with an ulcer on the inside of his lower lip that has been present for over six months and is slowing growing. He is a longstanding smoker and heavy drinker.

a) What is the most likely diagnosis?
b) How would you investigate this patient?
c) To which lymph nodes would this lesion drain?
d) The patient later develops a Horner's syndrome on the ipsilateral side. What is this and what could have caused it?
e) What is the TMN system and how is it used to define prognosis in patients such as this?

Answers

a) Squamous cell carcinoma (SCC) of the lip.
b) After a full history and examination the patient would require a CXR, CT or MRI of the neck, laryngoscopy and biopsy. There is a 10% risk of a second primary tumour being present at the same time (synchronous).
c) From the lip lymph drainage goes primarily to the submental and submandibular sites.

Lymph node site/region	Primary cancer site
Submental, submandibular	Lip, oral cavity, skin, salivary gland
Upper jugular	Oral cavity, oropharynx, larynx, nose, salivary gland
Mid jugular	Oral cavity, oro and hypopharynx, thyroid
Lower jugular	Oro and hypopharynx, larynx, cervical oesophagus, thyroid
Accessory nerve nodes	Nasopharynx, scalp
Supraclavicular	Breast, abdomen, thorax
Suboccipital	Skin
Parotid nodes	Skin, parotid

d) Horner's syndrome is the clinical picture of ptosis (drooping of the upper eyelid), miosis (constricted pupil) and anhydrosis (loss of sweating) of the cheek on the same side. It is due to metastatic lymph node invasion of the cervical sympathetic chain.
e) The system is used to stage the tumour to give an idea of prognosis based on the local extent of the tumour (T), nodal involvement (N) and presence of distant metastases (M).

Case 4

A 33-year-old woman has just returned to the ward after undergoing a thyroidectomy for a multi-nodular goitre. The nursing staff ask you to see her urgently as she appears to be having difficulty breathing and has developed a large swelling in her neck. Her observations are: pulse 117, blood pressure 100/52, respiratory rate 24, oxygen saturations on four litres is 91%.

a) What is the most likely cause for her distressing symptoms?
b) What is the appropriate immediate management of this patient?
c) What should you do next?

d) Twelve hours later you are called to see her again as she is complaining of numbness around her lips and her hands have gone into spasm. What is happening to her and what is the cause?

e) How should you treat this symptom?

f) What are the other potential complications of thyroidectomy?

Answers

a) The swelling in the neck that is causing respiratory embarrassment and is associated with hypotension and tachycardia is likely to be due to acute bleeding leading to the development of a haematoma that is confined within the wound and steadily leads to compression of the oesophagus, pharynx and trachea. This leads to difficulty in swallowing and respiratory distress.

b) The patient needs urgent intervention to free her airway. This means that the skin suture or staples must be removed and the wound opened to release the haematoma and relieve the pressure.

c) This remains a surgical emergency. Call the surgeon and anaesthetist immediately as the patient may need to return to theatre to stop any continued haemorrhage. In the meantime provide fluid resuscitation and make sure that the blood is cross-matched to replace the blood lost. Provide high flow oxygen, analgesia and try to reassure the patient and her family.

d) This is tetany and is caused by hypocalcaemia, which is due to the acute lack of parathyroid hormone. This is probably due to the inadvertent removal of or damage to the parathyroid glands during thyroidectomy. Any remaining parathyroid tissue may take some hours to days to produce adequate levels of parathyroid hormone to correctly manage calcium homeostasis.

e) The patient requires urgent calcium replacement which can be given both intravenously and orally. She will need close monitoring of her ionised calcium and appropriate replacement. She may also need vitamin D replacement to encourage oral absorption of the calcium supplements.

f) Other potential complications of thyroidectomy are hypothyroidism, infection and damage to or division of the recurrent laryngeal nerves, which supply the vocal cords. This can lead to hoarseness or stridor. Bilateral recurrent laryngeal nerve injury can cause airway obstruction as the neutral (paralysed) position of the cords is in the midline.

Case 5

A 50-year-old man presents to your clinic complaining of pain and a swelling under his jaw when he eats. This has been going on for several months and only affects the left side. The swelling appears when he eats and resolves after two to three hours. He has also noticed an unpleasant gritty taste in his mouth and can feel a lump at the base of his tongue on the left.

a) What is the most likely diagnosis?
b) What are the most common causes for this condition?
c) What are the potential complications of this condition?
d) Describe the investigation of this patient.
e) How would you manage this patient?

Answers

a) This is a typical history for a stone (calculus) in the duct of the submandibular gland on the left side. If the gland is partly blocked by the presence of a stone, when the gland is stimulated during mastication (particularly of sour foods such as lemon) the gland will swell. The most common glands affected by calculi are the submandibular glands as they produce 60% of saliva and the duct is long and runs in a slightly uphill course to the base of the tongue where stones can be palpated.

b) The most common causes are autoimmune diseases that lead to a dry mouth such as Sjogren's syndrome and systemic lupus erythromatosis or drugs such as anti-depressants and anti-cholinergic drugs.

c) The duct can become completely blocked and develop supra-added infection leading to a tense, hot and extremely painful submandibular swelling. The patient can become systemically unwell with a fever and raised white cell count. If the duct remains chronically blocked eventually the gland atrophies leading to decreased saliva production and aggravating the dry mouth symptoms.

d) After taking a history, the patient is examined using bimanual palpation of the floor of the mouth and cheek to feel along the course of the submandibular ducts and the parotid ducts for a palpable stone. Plain X-rays may reveal a radio-opaque calcium stone. A sialogram, where radio-opaque contrast is injected directly into the duct and an X-ray is taken, is the most appropriate investigation. It gives good images of the duct and the stone.

e) Simple measures such as advising the patient to drink plenty of water and keep well hydrated; sucking sour sweets, which encourages the flow of saliva and may stimulate expulsion of the stone, and massaging the salivary gland to clear thickened secretions will help. Change any medications which may be the cause and treat any underlying autoimmune disease. There are drugs available which stimulate saliva secretion such as anti-histamines or salagen. The stone may be removed by manual palpation and milking, or may need surgical removal.

Extended Matching Questions

EMQ 1

a. Lingual nerve
b. Trigeminal nerve
c. Carotid arteries
d. Superficial temporal artery
e. Pharynx
f. Facial nerve
g. Thoracic duct
h. Recurrent laryngeal nerve
i. Superficial temporal artery
j. Trachea

Select the important anatomical structure that is at most risk of iatrogenic injury during the following procedures:

1) Left hemithyroidectomy.
2) Excision of the submandibular gland.
3) Excision chemodectoma.
4) Superficial parotidectomy.
5) Excision biopsy left supraclavicular lymph node.
6) Excision of a branchial sinus.
7) Excision of a thyroglossal cyst.

Answers

1) h.
Hemithyriodectomy can lead to injury to the recurrent laryngeal nerve in its course inferior to the inferior thyroid vessels, middle thyroid vein and as it passes into the groove between the trachea and oesophagus.

2) a.
The lingual nerve is at risk during excision of the submandibular gland as it loops around the duct from above to lie medial to it.

3) c.
A chemodectoma (a carotid body tumour) arises in the bifurcation of the carotid artery between the internal and external carotid arteries.

173

4) f.
The facial nerve runs through the parotid gland separating it into deep and superficial parts.

5) g.
The thoracic duct lies just posterior to the left supraclavicular lymph node.

6) c.
The branchial sinus passes between the carotid arteries on its way to the pharynx, putting these vessels and the hypoglossal nerve which lies anterior to them at risk.

7) j.
The thyroglossal cyst lies in the midline anterior to the trachea, which may therefore be injured during resection.

EMQ 2

a. Grave's disease
b. Medullary carcinoma of the thyroid
c. Primary hypothyroidism
d. Pituitary failure
e. Primary hyperparathyroidism
f. Secondary hyperparathyroidism
g. Tertiary hyperparathyroidism
h. Lymphoma of the thyroid
i. Acute Hashimoto's thyroiditis

Select the appropriate diagnosis for the biochemical profiles given below:

	Thyroid stimulating hormone	T4	Anti-thyroid peroxidase antibody	Long acting thyroid stimulators	Calcium	Parathyroid hormone	Creatinine
1	N	H	H	N	N	N	N
2	L	L	N	N	N	N	N
3	N	N	N	N	H	H	H
4	N	N	N	N	H	H	N
5	N	N	N	N	L	H	H
6	L	H	N	H	N	N	N
7	H	L	N	N	N	N	N

(Key: N = normal, H = high, L = low)

Answers

1) i.
Antithyroid peroxidase antibodies are found in thyroid disease however they are particularly high in Hashimoto's thyroiditis (95% of patients). In the acute phase this condition causes the release of thyroxine from the inflamed gland leading to temporary hyperthyroidism, before it burns out to produce a primary hypothyroidism with high TSH and low thyroxine (T4) levels.

2) d.
In hypopituitarism, the deficiency may be of one or several hormones. Lack of TSH leads to hypothyroidism.

3) g.
Occasionally a patient with CRF overshoots the compensatory process and autonomously develops unnecessarily high PTH, with high calcium. This is tertiary hyperparathyroidism.

4) e.
Primary hyperparathyroidism is most often caused by a parathyroid adenoma (90% single, 10% all four glands are involved). These patients have a high parathyroid hormone (PTH) level and high calcium in the presence of normal renal function.

5) f.
Patients with chronic renal failure (CRF) have chronically high phosphate and low calcium which stimulates a secondary increase in PTH.

6) a.
High levels of long acting thyroid stimulator (LATS) are found in Grave's hyperthyroidism, i.e. high levels of total thyroxine (T4) with compensatory inhibited levels of thyroid stimulating hormone (TSH).

7) c.
In primary hypothyroidism there is inadequate thyroxine produced with compensatory elevated levels of TSH, whilst in pituitary failure (secondary hypothyroidism), the pituitary gland is unable to produce TSH, therefore the thyroid gland is not stimulated to produce thyroxine (T4), therefore levels of both are low or absent.

EMQ 3

a. Ranula
b. Melanoma
c. Dermoid cyst
d. Cystic hygroma
e. Basal cell cancer
f. Benign melanocytic naevus
g. Sebaceous cyst
h. Squamous cell cancer
i. Thyroglossal cyst
j. Branchial cyst

Select the most likely diagnosis from the choices given above:

1) A cystic mass commonly found in the posterior triangle of the neck caused by abnormal development and obstruction of the lymphatic system.
2) A congenital skin inclusion cyst.
3) Commonly presents in children and young adults as a cystic swelling in the anterior triangle of the neck and may form a fistulous opening along the anterior border of sternocleidomastoid.
4) A young woman presents with a pigmented macular papular lesion on her abdomen with an irregular edge which has recently increased in size and bleeds after a minor knock.
5) A 55-year-old man presents with a pigmented papule on his back which he has had for decades.
6) A midline cystic swelling in the neck that moves with swallowing and protrusion of the tongue.
7) An 80-year-old man presents with a 1 cm papular lesion on his forehead with a pearlescent sheen and ulcerated centre.

Answers

> **1) d.**
> A cystic hygoma is a lymph-filled cyst found in the posterior triangle of the neck which commonly presents in babies.
>
> **2) c.**
> A branchial cyst is a cystic swelling most commonly presenting in young adults and lies anterior to the anterior border of sternocleidomastoid.

A ranula is a retention cyst found in the floor of the mouth arising from the sublingual salivary glands.

3) j.
A dermoid cyst is a congenital inclusion of skin and appendages most commonly found at the medial and lateral angles of the eyebrows or the midline of the nose, neck and upper chest.

4) b.
A typical malignant melanoma presents with an irregular margin, variation in colour and depth and fragility making it prone to bleeding.

5) f.
A melanocytic naevus is a well circumscribed, pigmented macule or papule otherwise known as a mole.

6) i.
Thyroglossal cysts are cystic swellings found in the midline of the neck which move upwards on swallowing.

7) e.
BCCs are typically smooth with a pearlescent sheen and ulcerated centre. Whilst an SCC is also found in sun-damaged skin such as the hands, face and ears and appears as a small, firm erythematous plaque or nodule with indistinct margins that may become verrucous or ulcerated.

EMQ 4

a. Koebner phenomenon
b. Xanthelasmata
c. Keratoacanthoma
d. Marjolin's ulcer
e. Neurofibroma
f. Lentigo maligna
g. Alopecia
h. Lichenification
i. Bowen's disease
j. Warts

Select the most appropriate diagnosis for the definitions given below:

1) Carcinoma-*in-situ* that starts as a slow growing, non-invasive scaly red plaque, also known as intra-epidermal epithelioma, commonly found on the lower legs.
2) Skin thickening which leads to visibly exaggerated skin lines.
3) A proliferation of melanocytes that replaces the basal cell layer of the skin; commonly develops on the face in elderly women, rarely metastasises.
4) Hair loss.
5) When other skin conditions such as psoriasis, lichen planus, eczema, warts or vitiligo occurs in sites of scars or burns.
6) Yellow plaques commonly seen on the eyelids.
7) Infection of epidermal cells by human papilloma virus.
8) A benign tumour derived from peripheral nerve elements.
9) A fast-growing, benign, self-limiting papule plugged with keratin.
10) Squamous cell carcinoma that develops in long-standing unhealed wounds such as burns or chronic venous ulcers.

[Correct: 1) i., 2) h., 3) f., 4) g., 5) a., 6) b., 7) j., 8) e., 9) c., 10) d.]

Answers

The explanations are self-explanatory!

EMQ 5

a. Measure calcitonin
b. Surgical excision
c. Conservative management
d. Aspiration and injection sclerotherapy
e. Antibiotics and surgical drainage
f. Therapeutic radioactive iodine
g. Thyroidectomy
h. Chemotherapy

Select the most appropriate treatment option or investigation for the patients described below:

1) A 52-year-old man presents with a prominent sebaceous cyst on his scalp.
2) A 39-year-old man who had a thyroidectomy for medullary carcinoma 12 months ago.

3) A 16-year-old girl who has a small cystic hygroma and is terrified of the option of surgery.
4) A 33-year-old woman with a tender, red, hot swelling of the submandibular gland.
5) A 40-year-old woman who has recently undergone thyroidectomy for a papillary carcinoma.
6) A 70-year-old man with Stage IV lymphoma involving the thyroid gland.

Answers

1) b.
A sebaceous cyst is a benign, but often irritating lesion found in hair-bearing skin and is best managed by surgical excision.

2) a.
Measuring calcitonin levels can be used to monitor therapeutic efficacy and as a marker of recurrence of medullary carcinoma in patients who have undergone thyroidectomy.

3) d.
Aspiration and injection of a chemical agent that causes sclerosis (i.e. inflammation and fibrotic scarring of the cyst) is a good alternative to surgical excision for a cystic hygroma.

4) e.
Antibiotics and drainage is the treatment of choice.

5) f.
Papillary carcinoma is often multifocal and may spread to local lymph nodes. It is sensitive to radioactive iodine which is used as an adjunct to surgery to "mop up" any residual cancer cells.

6) h.
Disseminated lymphoma is treated with chemotherapy.

Chapter 8   Hernias

Ben Bannerjee and Gerard Stansby

Multiple Choice Questions

[Each single best answer (SBA) question comprises a stem and a number of answers. You are asked to decide which single item represents the best answer to the question.]

1. **Incisional hernias**

    a)   Are increased by post-operative wound infection
    b)   Can be prevented by use of a corset
    c)   Always require surgical correction
    d)   Are more common in thin patients
    e)   Can be avoided by using laparoscopic surgery

[Best Answer = a]

Explanation

The development of incisional hernias is multi-factorial and the causes broadly fall into two categories. Firstly, technical factors include post-operative haematoma or infection, bad closure technique or wrong suture material, the presence of stomas or drains and the choice of incision. Secondly, tissue factors including age, immuno-suppression (e.g. diabetes, jaundice, steroid therapy), obesity, malig-nant disease and malnutrition.

Laparoscopic surgery has its own incisional hernia that is the "port site hernia". Surgical correction is indicated for large or symp-tomatic hernias together with those at risk of obstruction or strangu-lation. Hernias not in these groups can be managed conservatively.

2. **Femoral hernias**

    a)   Are the predominant groin hernia presenting in women
    b)   Are more common in women than men
    c)   Have a low risk of obstruction

d) Can be felt as a cough impulse inferior and medial to the pubic tubercle
e) Should only be repaired if symptomatic

[Best Answer = b]

Explanation

> Although femoral hernias are more common in women than men, overall inguinal hernias are more common than femoral hernias in women. Due to the narrow femoral canal they are a high risk of obstruction and strangulation and should always be repaired. They are usually felt as a cough impulse over the femoral canal, which is inferior and lateral to the pubic tubercle.

3. **The inguinal canal**

   a) Contains the ovarian vessels in women
   b) Is normally obliterated after decent of the testicle
   c) Is bounded inferiorly by the inguinal ligament
   d) Allows the ureter to pass to the bladder
   e) Contains the blood supply to the penis

[Best Answer = c]

Explanation

> The inguinal canal is an oblique space passing between the musculo-aponeurotic layers of the abdominal wall transmitting the spermatic cord and testicular vessels from the retroperitoneum into the scrotum. It is short in the foetus and newborns. Anteriorly is the external oblique; posteriorly is the transversalis fascia; inferiorly the inguinal ligament; and superiorly the arching fibres of the internal oblique muscle. It additionally contains nerves (genital branch of genitofemoral and autonomic), lymphatics draining to the para-aortic nodes and the processus vaginalis. In women it contains the round ligament of the uterus.

4. **Concerning inguinal hernias one of the following statements is false**

   a) Can be caused by the failure of the processus vaginalis to obliterate
   b) Are more prominent during straining or coughing

c) Are usually direct hernias in infants
d) Are more common in men than women
e) Can extend into the scrotum

[Best Answer = c]

Explanation

> Indirect hernias are due to failure of the processus vaginalis to obliterate completely. This constitutes a congenital tendency to develop hernias and accounts for all inguinal hernias presenting in infancy. Patients complain of increased prominence during any manoeuvre that raises intra-abdominal pressure, e.g. straining, coughing or bending down. The male to female ratio is 10:1 and in extreme circumstances they can extend into the scrotum.

5. Umbilical hernias

a) In infants usually require surgery before school age
b) In the adult, are associated with obesity
c) Are usually painless
d) Are more common than inguinal hernias
e) Usually contain small bowel

[Best Answer = b]

Explanation

> Umbilical hernias are present in many neonates in minor degrees. They are only very rarely irreducible and most undergo spontaneous reduction in size with very few persisting beyond puberty. In the adult they are uncommon before 40 years old with an equal male female distribution. They occur less commonly than inguinal hernias. They are associated with obesity and often patients present with discomfort as they are often irreducible. They usually contain omentum although can also contain transverse colon or small bowel rarely.

6. **A rarer hernia which is more common in elderly women**

   a) Axillary
   b) Vertebral
   c) Obturator
   d) Ilio-psoas
   e) Scalene

[Best Answer = c]

Explanation

> Obturator hernias are rare hernias in elderly women in which small intestine herniates through the obturator canal in the lower part of the pelvis. They are difficult to diagnose and often present late due to this. They present with small bowel obstruction and pain on the inside of the thigh due to pressure on the obturator nerve.

7. **A strangulated hernia**

   a) Can be treated by reducing the hernia
   b) May be reducible
   c) Is usually painless
   d) Should be managed with early surgery
   e) Is more commonly observed in inguinal than femoral hernias

[Best Answer = d]

Explanation

> A strangulated hernia is one in which the blood supply of the contents of the hernia, has been compromised due to the narrowness of the neck. Once this occurs, gangrene of the bowel can set in. They are usually irreducible. It constitutes a surgical emergency and should be operated on as soon as possible. It occurs in femoral more than inguinal hernias due to the narrowness of the femoral canal.

8. An indirect inguinal hernia

a) Exits the inguinal canal lateral and superior to the pubic tubercle
b) Can be controlled by reducing the hernia and pressing on the deep ring
c) In females, can extend into the vaginal wall
d) Is less common when there is an undescended testicle
e) Has a lower incidence of obstruction when compared to direct hernias

[Best Answer = b]

Explanation

The superficial ring of the inguinal canal is medial and superior to the pubic tubercle. Indirect hernias enter the inguinal canal through the deep ring and as such are said to be controllable by pressure over that area after reduction of the hernia. In women inguinal hernias uncommonly extend into the labia majora. In childhood commonly and occasionally in adults, it is associated with undescended testicles. Indirect hernias do have a higher risk of obstruction due to their narrow neck. Direct hernias tend to have a broad neck (i.e. the defect in the transversalis fascia).

9. Direct inguinal hernias

a) Are associated with smoking or a chronic cough
b) Arise from a defect in the external oblique muscle
c) Are worse on lying flat
d) Occur frequently in women
e) Can cause urinary retention

[Best Answer = a]

Explanation

Direct inguinal hernias are due to a weakness in the transversalis fascia, medially behind the cord structures, in the inguinal canal. They are associated with COPD and smoking. They are usually relieved by lying flat and rarely occur in women (usually indirect).

10. An incarcerated hernia

a) Can be reduced with care
b) Is best managed conservatively
c) Occurs more frequently in incisional hernias
d) Can be associated with constipation
e) Is usually strangulated

[Best Answer = d]

Explanation

Incarcerated hernias are those that cannot be reduced. Early surgical intervention is usually indicated. They are uncommon in incisional hernias which are usually broad necked and reducible. Straining due to constipation can be a cause of incarceration as can the presence of cirrhosis with ascites.

11. One of the following is false concerning inguinal hernia repair

a) Can be performed under local anaesthetic
b) Can be complicated by urinary retention
c) Laparoscopic repair is indicated in bilateral or recurrent hernias
d) Rarely involves the insertion of a polypropylene mesh
e) Has a high mortality in cases that are strangulated

[Best Answer = d]

Explanation

Inguinal and femoral hernia repair can be performed under general or local anaesthesia. Emergency repairs are usually performed under general anaesthesia and have a higher mortality. Older methods involved the use of sutures for repair. Modern techniques nearly always involve the insertion of a mesh, particularly laparoscopic procedures which are commonly used for bilateral or recurrent hernias.

12. Hiatus hernia

a) Is caused by gastro-oesophageal reflux
b) Can pre-dispose patients to oesophageal cancer
c) Can be complicated by stricturing of the stomach
d) Is eased when patients lie flat
e) Is associated with a high oesophageal pH on monitoring

[Best Answer = b]

Explanation

Hiatus hernia is associated with, not caused by, symptoms of gastro-oesophageal reflux. This usually results in heartburn and is made worse by lying flat or bending or straining. Oesophageal pH monitoring reveals greater acidity, i.e. a lower pH. It can be complicated by recurrent oesophagitis with stricture formation in the oesophagus. It can also pre-dispose to Barrett's oesophagus which is a pre-malignant condition.

13. Parastomal hernia

a) Occur in more than 40% of stomas formed
b) Are of a lower incidence when the stoma is placed lateral to the rectus muscle
c) Are of a lower incidence in loop stomas
d) Do not cause intestinal obstruction
e) Are associated with obesity

[Best Answer = e]

Explanation

Parastomal hernias complicate approximately 10% of all stomas. Their incidence is decreased when the stoma is placed through the rectus muscle as opposed to the weaker flank musculature. Loop stomas involve making a defect in the abdominal wall for two bowel ends and as such have a higher hernia incidence as with obesity. They can cause obstruction of flow from the stoma and this is by no means rare.

14. One of the following is false concerning recurrent inguinal hernias

a) Can be due to bad surgical technique
b) Are a common occurrence
c) Can be caused by haematoma formation at the original surgery
d) Can be repaired laparoscopically
e) Repair can result in testicular atrophy on the same side

[Best Answer = b]

Explanation

Recurrent inguinal hernias are not common today. The use of prosthetic mesh to cause a fibrotic tissue reaction in the hernial orifice has reduced recurrence rates to 0.5% in elective hernia repair. When recurrences are found it can often be related to an inexperienced surgeon, sepsis, haematoma or the "missed" hernia (indirect recurrence after repair of a direct hernia). They can be repaired more safely and efficiently with laparoscopy as one does not need to dissect through the previous scar tissue. Re-do hernia surgery can disrupt the blood supply to the testicle resulting in either atrophy or infarction.

15. Complications following hernia surgery include

a) Loss of sensation to the ipsilateral side of the penis
b) Loss of sensation to the skin of the lower abdomen
c) Impotence
d) Recurrence of the hernia
e) Hydronephrosis

[Best Answer = d]

Explanation

Most hernia repairs have some degree of numbness in the skin following hernia repair usually inferior to the wound. The common nerves injured during repair are the ilioinguinal and genitofemoral nerves, which usually cause loss of sensation on the medial thigh or the scrotum. Impotence is not normally associated with hernia repair. Recurrence of the hernia can occur in 0.5% of cases and urinary retention is a common complication of hernia repair in elderly men.

Case Studies

Case 1

A 55-year-old postman presents complaining of an intermittent lump in the left groin associated with some aching. He is otherwise well. He is asking to be fitted with a truss.

a) What is the most likely diagnosis?
b) How would this be confirmed?
c) What are the potential complications?
d) What is a truss and do they have a place in the management of this condition?
e) What are the management options?

Answers

> a) A clear history of an intermittent lump in the groin is highly suggestive of a hernia. The most likely diagnosis here is of an inguinal hernia or possible a femoral hernia. An inguinal hernia may be direct or indirect but this cannot be assessed with absolute certainty by clinical examination.
>
> b) The diagnosis would be confirmed on clinical grounds based on the history and physical examination. It is usually best to stand the patient when looking for a small hernia. The other groin and the scrotum should also be examined. If identified the relationship of a hernia to the landmark of the pubic tubercle should be established (inguinal above and medial, femoral below and lateral). In doubtful cases imaging such as an ultrasound may be required to demonstrate a hernia.
>
> c) The complications of an inguinal hernia include irreducibility, bowel obstruction and strangulation.
>
> d) A truss is a specially made belt incorporating pads to put pressure in the groin to keep the hernia reduced. By pressing on the neck of the hernia they may increase the risk of strangulation and their use is not usually recommended.
>
> e) In an active patient experiencing symptoms an inguinal hernia should be repaired. This may be done by either open or laparoscopic surgery. In both types of surgery a nylon mesh is usually inserted to strengthen the posterior wall of the inguinal canal. Open repair is usually preferred for unilateral primary hernias.

Case 2

A 45-year-old obese man is going to undergo a Lichtenstein mesh repair for an inguinal hernia.

a) Would this be carried out under local or general anaesthetic.
b) What are the principles of the operation?
c) What would you advise him about heavy lifting and return to work post-operatively?
d) What potential complications would you discuss with him?

Answers

a) Open mesh repair (Lichtenstein repair) can be carried out under either general or local anaesthesia.
b) The operation involves:

  - opening the inguinal canal by dividing the external oblique aponeurosis
  - identify the hernia and separate from the spermatic cord
  - for indirect hernias open the sac and reduce its contents to the abdomen, then ligate and excise the sac (called "herniotomy")
  - for direct hernias with a broad neck the sac is usually just inverted not excised
  - suture mesh onto posterior wall of inguinal canal to strengthen it
  - repair external oblique and close wound.

c) The patient is able to return to work as soon as the wound is comfortable enough. There is no need to avoid heavy lifting subsequently. Once the mesh is incorporated in the tissues it will not be disrupted by lifting or heavy manual work.
d) As with any operation the patient should be warned of general complications of surgery and anaesthesia as well as specific complications. Specific complications of hernia repair include wound infection, pain due to sensory nerve entrapment and recurrence of the hernia. In older men urinary retention is also a relatively common complication.

Case 3

A thin 75-year-old lady is admitted with the acute onset of colicky abdominal pain, abdominal distension, vomiting and absolute constipation. She has had no previous abdominal surgery.

a) What is the likely diagnosis?
b) How would you manage her case initially?
c) She is found to have a small lump in the right groin on examination. What might this be?
d) How would this alter the management plan?

Answers

a) Clinically she is suffering with acute intestinal obstruction.
b) She will need to be resuscitated, and an intravenous infusion started as she is likely to be fluid depleted. Electrolyte abnormalities will need correcting. A nasogastric tube should be passed to decompress her stomach. Analgesia should be given.
c) This is likely to be a femoral hernia, which will be below and lateral to the pubic tubercle. If it is irreducible and tender it is likely to be the cause of her acute intestinal obstruction.
d) If she has a strangulated femoral hernia she will need to undergo emergency repair of this. This should be carried out as soon as possible to reduce the risk of the strangulated bowel undergoing infarction. Usually the operation will be done through a "high" incision and not by an incision over the hernia, so that the bowel can be fully inspected and a resection of any non-viable bowel can be carried out if needed.

Case 4

A three-week-old male child presents with a lump in the left side of the scrotum most obvious when the infant is crying. He seems otherwise well.

a) What are the possible diagnoses?
b) What is a patent processus vaginalis?
c) What are the indications for surgery?
d) If the lump was at or near the umbilicus what would the diagnosis be and how would this condition be managed.

Answers

a) The most likely diagnoses are either an inguinal hernia or an infantile hydrocoele. The full differential diagnosis should also include an incompletely descended testicle (which may co-exist with an infantile hernia), a femoral hernia or enlarged lymph nodes.

b) A patent processus vaginalis is a remnant of peritoneum which carries down into the scrotum from the abdomen with the descent of the testicle. It can be responsible either for fluid to develop around the testicle (hydrocoele) or for intra-abdominal contents to enter the scrotum (a hernia).

c) It is important to differentiate between hydrocoele and hernia as the management differs. Early surgery is usually recommended for hernia due to the high risk of obstruction/strangulation. In contrast spontaneous resolution of hydrocoeles is common and they are usually observed until at least three years of age.

d) The lump is likely to be an umbilical or paraumbilical hernia. Umbilical and paraumbilical hernias in children are quite common and are usually asymptomatic. Strangulation is rare. Most of these will close spontaneously before the age of four years old. Only those that persist beyond this age or are particularly large are repaired surgically.

Case 5

An 80-year-old man presents with an abdominal swelling six months after a successful aortic aneurysm repair. The swelling is most noticeable when he is asked to lift his head up from the bed when lying flat.

a) What is the most likely cause of this swelling?
b) Why do they occur?
c) What is the risk of complications developing?
d) How should it be managed?

Answers

a) This is most likely to be an incisional hernia.

b) An incisional hernia is one that occurs through a previous surgical wound. They occur when the deeper layers of a wound (usually muscle and fascia) come apart but the skin remains intact. This may be due to failure of the suture material used to close the wound, increased intra-abdominal pressures due to factors such as chronic cough, constipation or prostatism or to poor healing due to steroid therapy, malnutrition or malignancy. They are also more common in the elderly, diabetics and those who have suffered with post-operative wound infections.

c) Most incisional hernias are broad necked and the risk of strangulation is low. However, this is not always the case and they can cause bowel obstruction or strangulation.

d) Many asymptomatic incisional hernias in elderly patients can be managed conservatively. An elastic abdominal support may be helpful. If they do require repair then several surgical techniques have been described including laparoscopic repair. Most commonly the techniques currently used involve placing a nylon mesh over the defect to produce a tension free repair.

Extended Matching Questions

EMQ 1

a. Inguinal lymphadenopathy
b. Femoral hernia
c. Pantaloon hernia
d. Femoral artery aneurysm
e. Haematoma
f. Indirect inguinal hernia
g. Saphena varix
h. Undescended testes
i. Lymphocoele
j. Exostosis of the femoral head
k. Direct inguinal hernia

Choose the diagnosis from the list above, which most fits the case scenarios described below:

1) A 70-year-old man who is a chronic smoker with a BMI of 20, presents to the clinic with a lump in his left groin that he says appeared after a bad exacerbation of his chronic obstructive pulmonary disease.
2) A 39-year-old woman presents with a painless groin lump with a cough impulse. She reports that this has appeared after the birth of her third child (full term normal delivery). She has always had varicose veins following the birth of her first child.
3) A 24-year-old lady has venous surgery for the second time on her left leg including a further exploration of her groin. One week later she has a swollen erythematous groin wound with a tense swelling present. Her temperature is normal.
4) A mother brings her five-month-old infant, who is fit and well and achieving all milestones, with a painless lump in the right groin that increases in size when he cries.
5) A 40-year-old lady reports to A&E with severe pain in the right groin. On examination she has a tender irreducible lump in that groin. The lump is inferior and lateral to the pubic tubercle.

Answers

1) k.
Direct inguinal hernias are due to a weakening of the transversalis fascia layer of the abdominal wall. This is at its weakest in the medial half of the posterior wall of the inguinal canal. Such hernias are often precipitated by excessive straining or coughing.

2) g.
Often mistaken for a hernia, this lady has a saphena varix. She has established varicose veins and a saphena varix is an abnormal dilatation of the long saphenous vein in the groin. Usually a dilated long saphenous vein further down the leg can be felt.

3) i.
Lymphocoeles are a common complication of re-do varicose vein surgery, occurring in as many as 25% of cases. Due to damage to groin lymph vessels, they often settle spontaneously but can require percutaneous drainage. An alternative diagnosis is that this might be a haematoma(e).

4) f.
Indirect inguinal hernias are due to a persistence of the processus vaginalis embryologically. This can result in these hernias presenting from birth. They are usually treated with surgical repair, herniorraphy.

5) b.
Although femoral hernias are more common in women versus men, inguinal hernias remain the more common hernia in both groups. However, in this case the hernia anatomically arises from the femoral canal and is therefore a femoral hernia. These hernias are more prone to present acutely with irreducibility and strangulation of bowel contents of the sac.

EMQ 2

a. Carry out a Nissen Fundoplication
b. Advise a corset to be worn
c. Recommend for laparoscopic repair
d. Suggest repair under local anaesthetic
e. Use a prolene mesh to repair
f. Request a herniogram

g. Conservative management
h. Suggest repair under general anaesthesia
i. Refer for gastroscopy

Select the most appropriate option for the patients described below:

1) A 65-year-old smoker with COPD and angina complains of severe heart burn particularly when lying flat or bending or straining.
2) A 50-year-old man has a straightforward right inguinal hernia. He is thin.
3) An obese lady attends with vague but significant pain in the right groin on standing or straining. Examination fails to reveal anything.
4) A fit 45-year-old gentleman who has bilateral inguinal hernias.
5) A frail 93-year-old gentleman with a large ventral hernia who lives in a nursing home.

Answers

> **1) i.**
> This patient most likely has a hiatus hernia, however gastroscopy is indicated to rule out more sinister pathology.
>
> **2) d.**
> This patient should be, with appropriate consent and agreement, suitable for local anaesthetic repair. This approach is limited by the body habitus of the patient together with compliance during surgery under local anaesthesia.
>
> **3) f.**
> Determining diagnosis of groin lumps in obese patients can be fraught with difficulty. Where there is doubt, further imaging must be obtained such that surgical efforts can be directed appropriately. Herniography, ultrasound, CT and even MRI can be useful in this situation.
>
> **4) c.**
> Laparoscopic hernia repair is currently recommended for patients with bilateral inguinal hernias or a recurrent inguinal hernia.
>
> **5) g.**
> Ventral (epigastric) hernias are usually low risk in terms of potential for strangulation due to their broad neck. As such, conservative (palliative) treatment is indicated in this particular case due to the high risks of surgery and anaesthesia.

EMQ 3

a. Pubic tubercle
b. Transversalis fascia and conjoint tendon
c. Genitofemoral nerve
d. Dartos muscle
e. External oblique
f. Ilioinguinal nerve
g. Anterior superior iliac spine (ASIS)
h. Cremaster muscle
i. Femoral canal
j. Internal oblique

Select the most appropriate answer for the statements below:

1) The origin of the inguinal ligament.
2) The muscular covering of the spermatic cord.
3) Supplies sensation to the medial aspect of the upper thigh, the scrotum and the root of the penis.
4) Forms the posterior wall of the inguinal canal.
5) Forms the anterior aspect of the inguinal canal.

Answers

1) g.
The inguinal ligament originates from the ASIS and inserts into the pubic tubercle.

2) h.
The cremaster muscle surrounds the cord. It is a thin layer of skeletal muscle between the internal and external spermatic fascia. It is often poorly developed with only a few fibres present. Its function is to raise the testes to help maintain a constant temperature and aid spermatogenesis.

3) f.
The ilioinguinal nerve runs in part of the inguinal canal and can be damaged during inguinal hernia repair. It enters the canal directly by perforating the muscle and does not pass through the deep ring.

4) b.

The posterior wall is formed by the transversalis fascia and the conjoint tendon which is formed from the conjoined tendons of the internal oblique and transversus abdominus muscles.

5) e.

The external oblique muscle is the outermost of the abdominal muscles. It has muscular and tendinous parts. The tendinous part (the external oblique aponeurosis) forms the anterior wall of the inguinal canal. Its very lowest margin forms the inguinal ligament.

EMQ 4

a. Abdominal ultrasound
b. Intravenous urogram
c. Laparotomy
d. Plain abdominal film
e. Ultrasound scan
f. Conservative management
g. Routine hernia repair
h. Transfemoral angiogram
i. Emergency hernia repair
j. Diamorphine infusion

Select the most appropriate answer for the statements below:

1) A 20-year-old man presents with abdominal pain and vomitting. Examination reveals a tender, hard irreducible swelling in his right groin.
2) A 70-year-old man has a lump in his left groin. Examination reveals it to be hard and pulsatile.
3) A 45-year-old woman has a reducible left groin lump, with discomfort on straining or coughing.
4) A 64-year-old man with severe COPD, on home oxygen with ischaemic heart disease has a large reducible left inguino-scrotal lump.
5) A 35-year-old man presents with a hard craggy irreducible lump in his right groin. He gives a history of hot sweats and shivering at night.

Answers

1) i.
This young man has an incarcerated hernia with probable small bowel obstruction. After appropriate resuscitation he should undergo emergency repair of his hernia. The sac ought to be opened to carefully inspect the integrity of the small bowel in the sac and if necessary, necrotic segment resected.

2) e.
This patient most likely has an iliac or common femoral aneurysm. Initially this needs to be imaged with ultrasound to confirm the diagnosis.

3) g.
The patient needs routine hernia repair, as there are no signs suspicious of the hernia becoming incarcerated.

4) f.
This gentleman is unlikely to tolerate an operation even if carried out under regional or local anaesthesia. Therefore conservative measures must be applied if possible.

5) e.
This young man most likely has lymphoma and CT scanning will provide the quickest answer as to whether this is the case by demonstrating retroperitoneal lymphadenopathy. Testicular examination would be mandatory as this could also be a testicular tumour.

EMQ 5

a. Strangulated
b. Obstructed
c. Sliding
d. Incarcerated
e. Irreducible
f. Incisional
g. Hiatus hernia
h. Parastomal

i. Richter's hernia
j. Obturator hernia

Select the most appropriate diagnosis for the statements below:

1) A sick, elderly patient is taken to theatre with a femoral hernia, which is found to contain gangrenous small bowel.
2) A man attends one year after an open aneurysm repair complaining of a swelling in the midline of his abdomen.
3) At surgery a right inguinal hernia is found to contain the caecum outside the peritoneal sac which contains small bowel.
4) These type of hernias may be sliding, rolling or mixed and can cause pain worse on bending, stooping or at night on lying flat.
5) A thin elderly lady presents with intestinal obstruction and pain felt on the inner aspect of the thigh.

Answers

1) a.
A hernia containing gangrenous bowel has undergone strangulation — where the blood supply has been compressed at the neck of the hernia. This is more common in hernias with tight necks such as femoral hernias.

2) f.
Incisional hernias — through previous scars are relatively common. Factors leading to the development of an incisional hernia include obesity, old age, chronic cough or straining due to constipation or prostatism and wound infection.

3) c.
A sliding hernia is one which contains a partially extraperitoneal structure, such as the caecum on the right or the sigmoid colon on the left. Therefore, the sac does not completely surround all the contents of the hernia. The importance of this is that particular care must be taken when excising the sac, to avoid damaging the bowel.

4) g.
Hiatus hernias may either be sliding (85%), rolling (10%) or mixed (5%). Heartburn (reflux oesophagitis) is typically worse on bending forward and at night.

5) j.
This hernia occurs into the obturator foramen inside the pelvis and does not usually produce a palpable lump. It is most commonly seen in thin elderly women. Pressure on the obturator nerve gives rise to pain felt on the inner aspect of the thigh.

Chapter 9   Fluid Balance and Parenteral Nutrition

Ian Nesbitt and Joe Cosgrove

Multiple Choice Questions

[*Each single best answer (SBA) question comprises a stem and a number of answers. You are asked to decide which single item represents the best answer to the question.*]

1. The following is a normal serum biochemical value

a) Sodium: 129 mmol/l
b) Potassium: 4.9 mmol/l
c) Magnesium: 0.38 mmol/l
d) Phosphate: 0.45 mmol/l
e) Creatinine: 140 mmol/l

[Best Answer = b]

Explanation

> Normal (reference) values vary somewhat, but typical values are: normal range of sodium: 135–145 mmol/l, normal range of potassium: 3.5–5.0 mmol/l, normal range of magnesium: 0.70–1.00 mmol/l, normal range of phosphate: 0.80–1.44 mmol/l, normal range of creatinine: 60–110 μmol/l.

2. Normal (0.9%) saline

a) May cause acidosis
b) Preferentially expands the intracellular space
c) Is mainly excreted via sweat
d) Is isotonic with intracellular fluid
e) Contains 154 mmol/l each of sodium and bicarbonate

[Best Answer = a]

Explanation

> "Normal" (isotonic with extracellular fluid) or 0.9% saline contains 154 mmol/l of sodium and chloride ions in water at a pH of around 5.0. Large volume infusions of 0.9% saline cause a hyperchloraemic metabolic acidosis, as the addition of chloride anions leads the body to maintain electrochemical homeostasis through regulating (i.e. losing) other anions that includes bicarbonate. Like Hartmann's solution, normal saline is distributed mainly in the extracellular space following intravenous infusion and it is mainly excreted via the kidneys.

3. Regarding potassium

a) Hyperkalaemia is associated with prolonged vomitting/diarrhoea/diuretic use
b) Hyperkalaemia can be treated with insulin and glucose infusion
c) Hypokalaemia is associated with tall tented T waves on ECG
d) Acidosis causes hypokalaemia
e) Magnesium levels should be checked if hyperkalaemia persists

[Best Answer = b]

Explanation

> Prolonged vomitting causes a hypokalaemic metabolic alkalosis, since the body attempts to conserve acid by excreting potassium. Magnesium and potassium are also linked ions, so management of refractory hypokalaemia should include a search for low magnesium levels. Acidosis causes hyperkalaemia. Hyperkalaemia causes tall peaked T waves (and ultimately a sinusoidal ECG appearance). Rapid management includes a glucose insulin infusion — the insulin drives potassium into the intracellular space, and the glucose prevents hypoglycaemia. Magnesium levels should be checked if hypokalaemia persists.

4. Albumin

a) Freely crosses the capillary membrane
b) Freely crosses the glomerular membrane

c) Freely crosses the cell membranes
d) Serum albumin is a good indicator of nutritional state in hospitalised patients
e) Is found in lymphatic fluid

[Best Answer = e]

Explanation

Albumin is a large, electrically charged structure, so does not cross membranes easily. Small amounts leak through capillary membranes to enter lymphatic fluid. Pre-albumin is a better indicator of nutritional status than albumin.

5. With respect to crystalloids

a) Glucose 5% is isotonic
b) Hartmann's solution has a higher concentration of sodium than 0.9% saline
c) Glucose 5% has a lower pH than 0.9% saline
d) Hartmann's solution contains 100 mmol/l lactate anions
e) One litre of glucose 10% contains 10 g of glucose

[Best Answer = c]

Explanation

Glucose 5% is hypotonic (280 mOsmol/l). Sodium concentration in 0.9% saline is 154 mmol/l and 131 mmol/l in Hartmann's solution. pH of 0.9% saline is 5.0 and pH of glucose 5% is 4.0 Hartmann's solution contains lactate (30 mmol/l) that generates bicarbonate through hepatic metabolism. One litre of glucose 10% contains 100 g of glucose.

6. When managing post-operative fluid requirements

a) Hypotension may worsen acute renal failure
b) Fluid restriction is always needed in liver failure

c) A central venous pressure of 4 mmHg usually indicates hypovolaemia
d) Excessive gastrointestinal stoma losses can be adequately replaced by 4% dextrose 0.18% saline solution ("dextrose saline")
e) Urine output is not a good indicator of organ perfusion in post-operative surgical patients

[Best Answer = a]

Explanation

Hypotension and subsequent renal hypoperfusion worsens acute renal failure. Although patients with liver failure may have a normal or even elevated blood volume they are often functionally hypovolaemic, they may therefore require volume resuscitation. The cardiovascular picture of severe liver failure is similar to septic shock. Be cautious when interpreting CVP readings in isolation. They should be read in the context of the overall clinical picture of the patient. In addition to water, excessive gastrointestinal loss contains electrolytes. "Dextrose saline" is therefore inadequate if all losses are to be replaced. In the majority of surgical patients oliguria is a good initial marker for volume status, however it should (as with the CVP) be taken in the context of overall clinical picture, catheter obstruction and any pre-existing renal disease.

7. **A serum sodium concentration of 142 mmol/l and potassium of 6.2 mmol/l are likely with:**

a) Acute renal failure
b) Addison's disease
c) Furosemide treatment
d) Hypothyroidism
e) Diarrhoea

[Best Answer = a]

Explanation

Acute renal failure may cause elevated serum potassium requiring emergency management. Sodium may be low, normal or high. Hyponatraemia is a feature of Addison's disease (around 90% of cases; hyperkalaemia occurs in two–thirds of cases). Most diuretics are more commonly associated with hyponatraemia and hypokalaemia. Hypothyroidism is more likely to cause hyponatraemia and a high creatinine. Since large volumes of water and potassium are absorbed from the bowel, diarrhoea is a well-recognised cause of hypokalaemia.

8. **In the first 24 hours after major surgery**

   a) Sodium is retained
   b) Potassium is retained
   c) Metabolic rate is decreased
   d) Urinary nitrogen levels fall
   e) ADH secretion is reduced

[Best Answer = a]

Explanation

Sodium excretion is impaired after major injury. It is independent of sodium uptake and may last several days. Potassium excretion is increased. It peaks at approximately 24 hours and usually terminates within 48 hours. During the initial post-surgery period glucocorticoids, catecholamines and glucagons are secreted leading to protein catabolism and hence the metabolic rate is increased. Increases in protein catabolism result in increased urinary nitrogen levels. ADH secretion increases as part of the stress response.

9. **During the first hour of untreated acute blood loss of 15% of blood volume**

   a) Peripheral vascular resistance decreases
   b) Fluid shifts from interstitial fluid space to the intravascular space

c) Oliguria is mainly due to ADH secretion
d) Capillary permeability is reduced
e) Reticulocyte count increases

[Best Answer = b]

Explanation

> Sudden acute blood loss such as trauma or major post-operative haemorrhage causes intravascular volume depletion. Part of the initial compensation for this is "autotransfusion" of fluid from the extracellular space into the intravascular space, along with peripheral vasoconstriction. ADH secretion is increased, but oliguria also results from reduced renal perfusion and glomerular filtration. Capillary permeability often increases (as part of the inflammatory response), but not in the first hour. Likewise, the reticulocytosis in response to haemorrhage occurs after a longer delay.

10. Regarding blood for transfusion

a) Positive is the universal donor
b) Is leukocyte depleted in the UK
c) Packed red cells have a haematocrit of 45%
d) A bag (unit) of red cells contains 400 ml blood
e) Contains up to 60 mmol/l potassium

[Best Answer = b]

Explanation

> O negative is the universal donor group. Blood in the UK is now leukocyte depleted, partly to reduce the immune effects of blood transfusion, and partly as a precaution against transmission of prion disease. Each unit of red cells contains between 250–300 ml of red cell concentrate, with a haematocrit of 65%. Potassium leaks out of the stored red cells, so potassium concentrations increase with age of stored blood, reaching up to 30 mmol/l.

11. Regarding blood transfusion

a) Oxygen carriage is enhanced for several days due to depletion of 2,3 DPG levels
b) Donated blood can be stored for up to 82 days
c) Transfusion reaction due to ABO mismatch is rarely due to clerical errors
d) The chance of developing infection as direct consequence of transfusion is 1/10,000
e) Transfusion can cause immune-mediated respiratory failure

[Best Answer = e]

Explanation

> Blood can be stored for up to 42 days (in the UK — longer in some other countries) depending on the storage medium used. Screening of donor blood is highly efficient, so the risk of directly transmitted infection is negligible. Most severe transfusion reactions are due to clerical errors, frequently by attending junior staff. Stored blood has a different composition from fresh blood, including reduced levels of 2,3 diphosphoglycerate. This impairs (but does not eliminate) oxygen carriage and delivery for a variable period after transfusion, often several days. Blood and blood products can cause fluid overload, but also transfusion-related acute lung injury (TRALI) — an immune-mediated injury similar to non-cardiogenic pulmonary oedema.

12. Which of the following are untrue with regards to malnutrition?

a) Often occurs after admission to hospital
b) Micronutrient malnutrition is as important as protein energy malnutrition
c) Often continues after hospital discharge
d) Is common in hospital inpatients
e) Is the principle cause of anaemia in hospital

[Best Answer = e]

Explanation

Many patients are ill and malnourished prior to hospital admission, and despite adequate nutritional provision, continue to be malnourished during and after their hospital stay. Micronutrients (minerals, vitamins, and so on) are often important co-factors in healing processes, and deficiencies in these are as important as protein starvation. Anaemia in hospital patients is commonly multi-factorial, and although malnutrition is a contributing factor, usually the underlying disease process and overt/covert blood loss are more important in causing anaemia.

13. Regarding the gastrointestinal (GI) tract

a) Around two litres a day of fluid is normally secreted into the GI tract
b) Post-operative ileus affects mainly the small bowel
c) Absent bowel sounds are an absolute contraindication to enteral feeding
d) Metoclopramide is a prokinetic and strong antiemetic drug
e) Erythromycin is a prokinetic drug

[Best Answer = e]

Explanation

There is little correlation between the ability to absorb feed and the presence of bowel sounds. Normal bowel produces around eight litres a day of fluid, even in the post-operative period when ileus is common. Post-operative ileus affects mainly the stomach (gastroparesis) and colon. Metoclopramide is a poor antiemetic, but enhances gastric emptying (mediated via motilin receptors). Erythromycin is a prokinetic as well as an antibiotic, with an action mainly at the proximal small bowel.

14. Removal of the distal two metres of small bowel can lead to:

a) Constipation
b) Steatorrhoea
c) Osteoporosis

d) Iron deficiency

e) Microcytic anaemia

[Best Answer = c]

Explanation

The terminal ileum is involved in the enterohepatic circulation. This includes bile acids, vitamin B12, and fat soluble vitamins (including vitamin D). Inadequate absorption of these can result in osteoporosis, anaemia, and diarrhoea (due to colonic irritation by bile acids). A much greater length of small bowel resection is required to cause general malabsorption and steatorrhoea. Iron is principally absorbed in the proximal small bowel and so an iron-deficient picture is unlikely.

15. Consequences of total parenteral nutrition (TPN) include

a) Pancreatitis

b) Altered gut flora

c) Reduced mortality after major surgery

d) Reduced gut permeability

e) Hypoglycaemia

[Best Answer = b]

Explanation

TPN involves delivering all the nutritional requirements by a venous catheter. Since the gut is not as active as normal, villous atrophy occurs, and the gut becomes more permeable to various substances. Additionally, the normal gut flora is altered. Although TPN can deliver adequate nutrition, the impact of this treatment on outcome after surgery is unclear, with little difference in mortality rates compared to enteral feeding. There is no association with pancreatitis. TPN solutions often cause hyperglycaemia.

Case Studies

Case 1

A 66-year-old man develops tachycardia, hypotension and respiratory distress three hours after the difficult insertion of an intravenous chemotherapy (Hickman) line under general anaesthesia. Examination shows high jugular venous pulse, central trachea, equal air entry bilaterally, SpO_2 92% (breathing room air), heart rate 130 bpm, Blood pressure 85/45, cold peripheries. Chest X-ray is not available.

a) What is the most likely clinical diagnosis?
b) What are three other possible diagnoses?
c) What is your immediate management?
d) What other investigations should you request?
e) What is the definitive treatment?
f) What CXR appearances would you expect to see with this problem?

Answers

a) Cardiac tamponade. A central line may erode or perforate the thin right atrial wall. Since this is within the pericardial reflection, blood tracks out into the pericardium, causing cardiac tamponade.

b) Tension pneumothorax, cardiac failure, pulmonary embolus. The high JVP with signs of circulatory failure helps differentiate from hypovolaemia, while the central trachea and equal air entry reduce the possibility of tension pneumothorax as the correct diagnosis (although tracheal deviation is a late sign of tension pneumothorax, and asymmetric air entry can be difficult to detect in a noisy ward environment).

c) Oxygen, good intravenous access and cautious fluid boluses, and get experienced help.

d) Chest X-ray, echocardiography, ECG.

e) Pericardiocentesis (preferably under ultrasound control).

f) Cardiac tamponade classically shows a globular heart on CXR, although frequently, the appearances are non-diagnostic. The value of a CXR is to exclude a different pathology (e.g. pneumothorax) or aid in confirming the clinical diagnosis (e.g. malposition of Hickman line tip). Pulmonary embolism may also be difficult to distinguish clinically from cardiac tamponade. Cardiac tamponade is a difficult and often missed diagnosis.

Case 2

A 48-year-old obese female with Type II diabetes (requiring drug treatment) undergoes an open cholecystectomy and intra-operative cholangiogram. She is prescribed intravenous saline at 40 ml/hr post-op. and diclofenac as part of her post-operative analgesic regime.

	Hb (g/dl)	WCC (× 1012/l)	Plt (× 1012/l)	Na (mmol/l)	K (mmol/l)	Urea (mmol/l)	Creatinine (mmol/l)
Pre-operative blood results:	13.4	9.1	320	139	4.9	5.4	86
Post-operative (day 2) blood results:	10.1	22.4	158	134	3.9	10.2	164

a) What is the most likely clinical diagnosis?
b) List four potential precipitants for such a diagnosis.
c) What is your immediate management?
d) What other bedside measurement can confirm your diagnosis?
e) What substances should be avoided/minimised in the post-operative period?
f) What drugs can reduce the incidence of contrast-associated renal dysfunction?

Answers

a) Acute renal failure (probably ATN). A rising urea and creatinine in the context of known causal factors makes acute renal failure the most likely diagnosis in this case.

b) Hypovolaemia, non-steroidal drugs, radiocontrast agent, sepsis. Metformin is also a possible contributing factor. The most likely precipitant is hypovolaemia (40 ml/hr is an inadequate replacement regime). Contributing factors include non-steroidal analgesics (such as diclofenac), pre-existing renal disease (as is common in diabetics — even with normal urea and electrolytes), hypoglycaemic agents such as metformin, and radiocontrast. In this case, radio-contrast agent is a less likely contributor, since the relatively small volumes used for a cholangiogram are not given intravenously.

c) ABC approach, with emphasis on rehydration — establish adequate circulating blood volume and perfusion pressure. Ongoing management depends on the patient's response to this.

d) Measure urinary electrolytes and osmolarity. In renal failure, the kidneys cannot re-absorb sodium, so causing a high (traditionally > 40 mmol/l) urinary concentration along with poor concentrating ability (osmolarity < 400 mOsm/kg). In hypovolaemic patients with adequate renal function, the urine is concentrated (urinary osmolarity traditionally > 500 mOsm/kg), with good sodium re-absorption (urinary sodium < 20 mmol/l). Diuretics invalidate this test and, frequently, are used by inexperienced staff as a (usually inappropriate) treatment for oliguria.

e) Nephrotoxins such as aminoglycosides, non-steroidal agents. Patients with renal dysfunction should avoid other nephrotoxins or have doses of many drugs reduced appropriately (the British National Formulary has an appendix detailing this).

f) N-acetyl-cysteine and sodium bicarbonate. There is some weak evidence that N-acetyl cysteine or sodium bicarbonate can reduce the incidence of post-radiocontrast renal failure when added to adequate volume loading. This is especially relevant for vascular and cardiac patients undergoing angiography.

Case 3

A 60-year-old man with gallstone pancreatitis returns to your ward after 35 days in the intensive care unit. He has a central line for TPN, two abdominal drains for irrigating the pancreatic bed, and a central line for i.v. access and blood sampling (since peripheral access is poor). Two days later, he develops hypotension, tachycardia, pyrexia, hypoxaemia, and confusion.

a) What is the most likely diagnosis?
b) What are three other possible diagnoses?
c) What investigations will be most useful?
d) What is your immediate management?
e) Should the central line be removed?
f) Should the TPN line be removed?

Answers

a) Sepsis from the TPN or central line.
b) Sepsis from another site (especially intra-abdominal), ongoing SIRS from pancreatitis, pulmonary embolism.

c) Blood cultures and full blood count. A chest X-ray and ECG will help exclude other diagnoses. Imaging of his abdomen is also required — probably ultrasound in the first instance, although a CT scan may be a more definitive investigation.

d) Remember ABC. Blood cultures, fluid replacement, and antibiotics.

e) Ideally, a suspected infected intravascular catheter should be removed, but when a line tip is cultured, many will not actually be infected. The decision to remove the line will depend on the exact clinical picture — especially the difficulty of replacing central lines and how unwell the patient is. Many line-related infections settle with removal of the line, but empiric antibiotics are frequently prescribed. A complex patient like this should be discussed with the microbiologists, since they have probably been treated with multiple courses of antibiotics already, and may have atypical organisms present. Fungal sepsis is increasingly a problem in complicated long-stay patients, and it may be appropriate to start antifungal prophylaxis even if appropriate cultures are negative.

f) If one intravascular catheter is infected, it is likely that all the other lines are infected or colonised too, and they should all be changed.

Case 4

A 60-year-old man with small bowel obstruction develops hypoxaemia and respiratory distress four hours after uneventful insertion of a nasogastric tube (NGT). His chest X-ray is shown below.

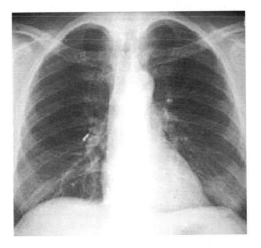

a) Is the respiratory distress likely to be related to the insertion of the tube?
b) How should placement of such a tube be confirmed in a ward setting?
c) Outline your initial management of the patient.
d) Are antibiotics indicated?
e) Which lung is typically involved, and why?
f) Should TPN be commenced immediately if nasogastric insertion is unsuccessful?

Answers

a) Yes — the chest X-ray shows the NGT in the right lung field. The path of the NGT is difficult to follow (this is often the case, especially with fine bore tubes), but the metal tip can be seen in the right mid zone beside the pulmonary vessels.

b) Test the aspirate with pH indicator paper and do a chest X-ray. NGT placement has traditionally been confirmed using litmus paper and the "whoosh" test (air is rapidly injected through the NGT while listening over the epigastrium). Neither method is infallible and a number of patients die each year from misplaced NGT. Recommended practice is that NGT position is confirmed using CXR and pH indicator paper testing of aspirate (more specific than litmus paper).

c) ABC approach, with removal of NG tube.

d) Not routinely. The initial chest X-ray changes of aspiration are often due to a sterile pneumonitis, which may not actually become infected. Many authorities suggest reserving antibiotics for proven infections only.

e) Right lung. The right main bronchus is less steeply angled than the left.

f) No. Several further attempts at NGT insertion are probably appropriate depending on the exact clinical circumstances (e.g. patient cooperation, trauma caused by NGT insertion, indication for insertion). Several days without feeding are unlikely to be detrimental for most patients, and TPN is not risk free — both from catheter insertion and from the feed itself, so TPN is not an immediate concern.

Case 5

A 58-year-old non-insulin dependent (Type II) diabetic is referred with a four-day history of vomitting and diarrhoea with abdominal pain and increasing drowsiness. She has been unable to take any of her normal medications. Abdominal examination is unremarkable. Initial tests show the following: blood pH 7.35;

blood glucose 44 mmol/l; sodium 153 mmol/l; potassium 5.1 mmol/l; urea 23 mmol/l; creatinine 152 mmol/l. Urine: glucose ++, no ketones.

a) What is the diagnosis?
b) What are the characteristic biochemical abnormalities of this illness?
c) What are three common precipitants for this illness?
d) What neurological complications occur with this disease?
e) What potential complications require prophylaxis?
f) What are appropriate initial replacement fluids?

Answers

a) Hyperosmolar non-ketotic coma (HONC/HONK), also called hyperosmolar hyperglycaemic non-ketotic coma (HHNC). Abdominal symptoms are not always due to a surgical cause. HONC is usually seen in adult onset diabetics. It is frequently precipitated by a non-specific acute illness, although pneumonia, urosepsis and myocardial infarction are common causes. Marked dehydration is a common feature. Abdominal pain can also occur (although it is more common with diabetic ketoacidosis).

b) Hyperglycaemia, hyperosmolarity, and the absence of significant ketosis. Other derangements are more variable. Pre-renal impairment can also cause high urea and creatinine.

c) Acute myocardial infarction, infection, gastrointestinal bleeding. In many cases, the precipitating cause is unknown.

d) Coma is uncommon in HONC, but a wide range of neurological abnormalities is possible and common ranging from non-specific confusion and drowsiness to focal abnormalities or seizure activity.

e) DVT and PTE are common complications of HONC and these patients should have thromboembolic prophylaxis. They are also at high risk of myocardial ischaemia.

f) Normal saline. Fluid deficits are often very large (many litres) in HONC. Despite the high serum sodium, aggressive replacement with normal saline initially is reasonable, followed by dextrose saline as the patient improves. Insulin is often required if blood glucose is slow to fall with fluid replacement only. Although serum potassium may be high initially, total body potassium is frequently depleted, and replacement usually required. Frequent monitoring of clinical response and laboratory values is necessary to gauge response to treatment.

Extended Matching Questions

EMQ 1

a. Diuretic therapy
b. Diabetes insipidus
c. Acute tubular necrosis
d. Artefact
e. SIADH (secretion of inappropriate ADH)
f. Iatrogenic
g. Diabetes mellitus

Match the most likely diagnosis with the biochemical disorder:

1) A 48-year-old man with polyuria in a psychiatric hospital awaiting electroconvulsant therapy.
2) A 14-year-old girl with recent onset polydypsia admitted with suspected appendicitis.
3) A 70-year-old man with oliguria two days after emergency aortic aneurysm surgery.
4) A 68-year-old woman with confusion and hyponatraemia (129 mmol/l) three days after hip surgery.
5) A 73-year-old with asymptomatic hyponatraemia (129 mmol/l). Admitted for resection of small cell carcinoma of the lung.
6) A 73-year-old hypertensive patient admitted for elective bowel surgery. Hyponatraemia (130 mmol/l) discovered on routine investigations.

Answers

1) b.
Various psychiatric drugs (especially lithium) are associated with nephrogenic diabetes inspidus.

2) g.
Diabetes mellitus commonly presents in teenage years, and is a recognised non-surgical cause of an acute abdomen.

3) c.
Emergency aortic aneurysm repair is associated with a high incidence of renal failure post-operatively. Acute tubular necrosis is the most common form of this.

4) f.

Symptomatic hyponatraemia within a couple of days of surgery is suggestive of inappropriate intravenous fluids — especially excessive volumes of dextrose.

5) e.

Asymptomatic hyponatraemia is associated with the syndrome of SIADH, often due to small-cell lung cancer.

6) a.

Asymptomatic hyponatraemia is a common side effect of diuretics — used to treat hypertension.

EMQ 2

a. Diabetes mellitus
b. Diabetes insipidus
c. Acute tubular necrosis
d. Artefact
e. Iatrogenic
f. SIADH
g. Diuretic therapy

Match the most likely diagnosis with the biochemical disorder. In each case, the patient is a 70 kg, 50-year-old man two days following the procedures specified in the table:

Q.	Procedure	Sodium (mmol/l)	Potassium (mmol/l)	Urea (mmol/l)	Creatinine (μmol/l)	Bicarbonate (mmol/l)	Glucose (mmol/l)
	(Normal values)	(135–146)	(3.5–5.0)	(2.5–6.7)	(60–120)	(22–30)	(4.5–5.6)
1	Emergency aortic valve replacement	135	5.0	10	300	15	4.3
2	Biopsy of neck lymphoma	129	5.0	7.7	100	24	4.3
3	Elective hip replacement	109	2.1	1.8	44	12	14
4	Craniotomy for meningioma	152	3.9	18	140	23	4.3
5	Elective varicose vein stripping	131	3.4	6.8	100	26	5.0
6	Elective inguinal hernia repair (patient stable)	136	8.7	5.5	106	26	6.1

Answers

1) c.

ATN causes a rapid increase in urea and creatinine, along with a metabolic acidosis (low bicarbonate). The potassium is at the upper end of normal range, but can sometimes remain relatively normal even with severe renal impairment. Emergency major surgery carries a high risk of renal dysfunction post-operatively (this is multifactorial — due to a combination of hypotension, sepsis, hypoxia, pre-existing renal impairment in elderly, drugs, etc.)

2) f.

Lymphoma is another disease associated with SIADH. Excess infusion of 5% dextrose may also cause hyponatraemia, but is less likely to be associated with a high urea.

3) d.

Multiple grossly abnormal values in a sample should raise suspicions of an artefact or iatrogenic cause, especially if the clinical situation makes abnormal results unlikely. The likely cause is that the blood was taken from the arm in which a drip was running.

4) b.

Diabetes insipidus is a recognised complication of head injury and brain surgery, although many cases are idiopathic. The uncontrolled diuresis leads to hypernatraemia, uraemia, and can even cause pre-renal renal failure.

5) g.

Many diuretics impair sodium retention and increase potassium excretion by the kidneys. A mild hypokalemia and hyponatraemia commonly results.

6) d.

A haemolysed sample of blood often has a high potassium (and high bilirubin), but is otherwise unremarkable. Often, the laboratory result will simply state "haemolysed" rather than values for potassium and bilirubin. If in doubt repeat the test.

EMQ 3

a. Vitamin B12 deficiency
b. Hypocalcaemia
c. Vitamin C deficiency
d. Hypokalaemia
e. Hyperkalaemia
f. Hypomagnesaemia
g. Hypophosphataemia

Match the most appropriate biochemical disorder with the symptom or sign:

1) A 79-year-old with partial gastrectomy 40 years ago, admitted for investigation of anaemia, ataxia and weakness.
2) Collapsed patient one week post-bowel surgery with Torsades de pointes on defibrillator screen.
3) A 52-year-old woman with new onset of peripheral paraesthesia two days after neck surgery.
4) A 60-year-old patient with vomitting and diarrhoea due to bowel obstruction.
5) A 63-year-old four days following bilateral ureteric obstruction during emergency pelvic surgery.
6) A 76-year-old patient developing peaked or "tented" T-waves on ECG during surgery.

Answers

1) a.
Pernicious anaemia may develop following gastrectomy. Vitamin B12 deficiency can cause subacute combined degeneration of the spinal cord.

2) f.
Torsades de pointes is a form of ventricular fibrillation that has a specific treatment — magnesium.

3) b.
A recognised complication of parathyroidectomy is hypocalcaemia-causing peripheral paraesthesia. Inadvertent parathyroidectomy may occur during thyroid surgery.

4) d.

Vomitting causes loss of hydrogen ions. In an attempt to conserve them, the body excretes potassium instead. Large bowel fluid contains a high potassium concentration. Vomitting and diarrhoea can cause refractory hypokalaemia.

5) e.

Acute obstructive nephropathy causes acute renal failure. One of the signs of this is hyperkalaemia.

6) e.

Hyperkalaemia can cause peaked or "tented" T-waves on ECG trace and asystole.

EMQ 4

a. Five per cent dextrose
b. Fifty per cent dextrose
c. Packed red cells
d. Hetastarch
e. Citrated sodium lactate (Hartmann's solution)
f. Ten per cent mannitol
g. Water for injection

Match the most appropriate intravenous fluid with the principal desired outcome:

1) Treatment of stage I haemorrhage.
2) Treatment of stage IV haemorrhage.
3) Expansion of total body water.
4) Expansion of extracellular space.
5) Treatment of hypoglycaemia.
6) Reduction in intracranial pressure.

Answers

1) e.

Stage I haemorrhage (less than 15% blood volume — c700 ml) can be managed without blood transfusion in many cases. Oral fluids alone may be adequate replacement, although generally, a crystalloid like Hartmann's solution is used peri-operatively.

2) c.
Stage IV haemorrhage is 40% or more loss of blood volume and is often immediately life threatening.

3) a.
Five per cent dextrose is metabolised to water — which distributes rapidly throughout the total body compartment.

4) e.
Crystalloids like Hartmann's or normal saline distribute rapidly across the capillary membrane to fill intravascular and interstitial compartments — the extracellular space.

5) b.
Small volumes of concentrated dextrose (20% or 50%) is most commonly used to treat hypoglycaemia.

6) f.
Mannitol is an osmotic diuretic. After an initial expansion of the intravascular space, it causes a reduction in intravascular and intracerebral volumes.

EMQ 5

a. Acute necrotising pancreatitis (ANP)
b. Short bowel syndrome following extensive abdominal surgery
c. Posterior circulation stroke with bulbar dysfunction
d. Proximal small bowel fistula after duodenal perforation
e. Patient with central vein stenosis and a stenosing oesophageal carcinoma
f. Left hemicolectomy patient, three days post-operatively

Match the disease process with the most appropriate form of feeding:

1) Total parenteral nutrition (TPN) via a central venous catheter.
2) Peripheral parenteral nutrition.
3) Percutaneous enterogastrostomy (PEG).
4) Nasogastric tube (NGT).
5) Oral feeding.
6) Feeding jejunostomy.

Answers

1) b.
Short bowel syndrome is an indication for TPN.

2) e.
Peripheral PN is a useful supplement if dysphagia is sufficient to make oral intake inadequate, and central venous access difficult.

3) c.
PEG insertion can reduce pulmonary aspiration following a cerebrovascular accident that causes bulbar dysfunction.

4) a.
Enteral nutrition may improve outcome in ANP and many such patients can attain satisfactory feeding with NGT feeding. A post-pyloric feeding tube would be indicated if not.

5) f.
Most left hemicolectomy patients should be eating by three days post-operatively.

6) d.
Feeding distal to a small bowel fistula can be achieved with a jejunal tube.

Chapter 10   Vascular Surgery

Gerard Stansby and Ben Bannerjee

Multiple Choice Questions

[*Each single best answer (SBA) question comprises a stem and a number of answers. You are asked to decide which single item represents the best answer to the question.*]

1. **Vascular claudication**

   a) Causes limping on walking
   b) Is usually felt in the foot at night
   c) Usually involves the thigh or buttock
   d) Is usually managed non-surgically
   e) Is a reason to be on anticoagulants

[Best Answer = d]

Explanation

> Claudication does not cause limping (although it comes from the Latin word for limping). It is most often felt in the calf muscles but can affect the thigh or buttock depending on the level of the arterial occlusion. Vascular rest pain, not claudication, is felt in the foot or toes. Most claudicants are managed non-surgically with reduction of vascular risk factors. This includes the use of antiplatelet agents but not usually anticoagulants.

2. **Ankle brachial pressure index (ABI)**

   a) Is measured using a Duplex scanner
   b) May be spuriously low in diabetics
   c) Is usually < 0.9 in claudicants
   d) Is calculated using systolic and diastolic pressures
   e) Is typically > 0.5 in patients with vascular rest pain

[Best Answer = c]

Explanation

> ABI is easy to measure as it requires only a hand-held Doppler probe (not a Duplex machine) and a sphygmomanometer. Only systolic pressures are used to calculate the ABI. Typically an ABI < 0.9 is regarded as abnormal and in critical ischaemia (rest pain) it is usually < 0.5 or unrecordable. In diabetics the ABI may be spuriously high because of calcification in the distal vessels which prevents them from being compressed by the sphygmomanometer cuff around the calf.

3. Chronic ankle ulcers

a) Are usually due to arterial disease
b) Should always be treated with compression bandaging
c) Should be biopsied if not healing
d) Are more common below the medial malleolus
e) Should be treated with topical antibiotics

[Best Answer = c]

Explanation

> The majority of chronic ankle ulcers are due to chronic venous disease (>70%), other causes are arterial disease (c. 10%), and mixed arterial and venous disease (c.10%). Venous leg ulcers are usually above the medial malleolus and are treated with compression but this may be harmful in arterial disease, which should be excluded by checking the ABI. Rarer causes include vasculitis and rheumatoid arthritis. Long standing ulcers may undergo malignant change (called a Marjolin's ulcer). Chronic non-healing ulcers should therefore be biopsied.

4. Carotid body tumours

a) Are usually malignant
b) Are usually diagnosed by biopsy
c) Are typically bilateral

d) Can be moved laterally but not vertically

e) Are usually treated with radiotherapy

[Best Answer = d]

Explanation

> Only about 5% of carotid body tumours are malignant and 5%–10% are bilateral. The diagnosis can usually be made on CT or MRI scan and biopsy is not normally needed. A carotid body tumour is pulsatile and may on occasion feel expansile, although it is not truly expansile. The mass is usually mobile from side to side but not vertically because it is restricted by the carotid bifurcation, which does not move up and down. Often a high-flow bruit over the tumour can be heard. Ideally they are treated by surgical resection and radiotherapy is reserved for inoperable or malignant cases.

5. **Aortic aneurysms**

a) Should be repaired as early as possible to prevent rupture

b) Arise most commonly in the infra-renal abdominal aorta

c) Are associated with hyperthryroidism

d) When ruptured are associated with an overall 30%–50% mortality

e) Are usually associated with aneurysms of the popliteal artery

[Best Answer = b]

Explanation

> Aneurysms should normally only be repaired if greater than 5.5 cm in size or symptomatic. If smaller they should usually just be followed up with regular ultrasound scans, as the risk of rupture is low. They are associated with all the major risk factors for atherosclerosis in general including hypertension but not hyperthyroidism. They most commonly affect the aorta below the renal arteries. Popliteal aneurysms are important but are associated with only a minority of abdominal aneurysms. Ruptured aneurysms have a >80% mortality overall because two-thirds die before reaching the hospital where the mortality is then 30%–50%.

6. Acute lower limb ischaemia

a) Should be treated by embolectomy
b) Is characterised by the presence of micro-infarcts on the foot
c) Is initially managed with heparin intravenously and observation
d) Requires immediate referral to a vascular surgeon
e) Is defined as an ankle brachial pressure index of less than 0.5

[Best Answer = d]

Explanation

Acute lower limb ischaemia is mostly due to embolism (often from the heart) or thrombosis at the site of pre-existing atheroma. For embolus, surgery is usually embolectomy using a Fogarty catheter but for thrombosis, an emergency bypass may be needed. It causes impairment of muscle and nerve function. (Remember the 6 "P's" — pain, pallor, pulseless, paralysis, paraesthesiae and perishing cold!) Infarcts are a late sign. All cases should be given heparin initially to prevent further extension of the thrombosis but observation is not correct. They should also be referred urgently for vascular surgery as the limb may be lost in three to six hours without intervention. It is not defined by the ABI, which will usually be unrecordable in acute ischaemia.

7. Vasculitis

a) Can be a complication of rheumatoid arthritis
b) Is secondary to atherosclerosis
c) In Henoch-Schonlein purpura is more commonly observed in adults
d) Is usually associated with an elevated cholesterol
e) Can be treated with non-steroidal anti-inflammatory agents

[Best Answer = a]

Explanation

Vasculitis means inflammation of blood vessels. The presentation varies enormously depending on which vessels are mainly involved. It may be primary or secondary to other conditions such as rheumatoid arthritis but not atherosclerosis. Markers of inflammation such as CRP are usually raised but not necessarily cholesterol. Henoch-Schonlein purpura occurs mainly in children. Vasculitis is usually treated with corticosteroids or immunosuppressive agents.

8. **Carotid artery stenosis due to atheroma**

a) Is diagnosed by the presence of a bruit over the lateral aspect of the neck
b) Causes approximately 50% of all strokes
c) Can be managed with surgical endarterectomy
d) Can be managed with thrombolysis
e) Can cause a haemorrhagic stroke by producing emboli

[Best Answer = c]

Explanation

A carotid bruit, although suggestive, is not diagnostic for significant internal carotid artery disease. Specific diagnosis requires imaging, most commonly by colour duplex ultrasound scanning. Narrowing at the origin of the internal carotid artery is the cause of about 15% of strokes and if symptomatic is usually treated by the surgical procedure of carotid endarterectomy. Strokes are caused either by emboli from the stenosis or by limitation of flow due to thrombosis of the internal carotid. More recently some cases are also being treated by percutaneous balloon angioplasty and stenting. Thrombolysis is increasingly being used for acute non-haemorrhagic (thrombotic or embolic) stroke but does not treat a carotid stenosis.

9. **The major risk factors for peripheral occlusive arterial disease include**

a) The female sex
b) Premature menopause
c) HDL greater than 1.0 mmol/l
d) Diabetes insipidus
e) Hypertension

[Best Answer = e]

Explanation

Peripheral arterial disease is associated with the same risk factors as coronary disease. The most important are smoking and diabetes mellitus (not insipidus). HDL-cholesterol is protective — the higher the HDL the less the risk.

10. Iliac vein thrombosis

a) Is often caused by direct malignant involvement of the vein
b) Is a common cause of varicose veins
c) May cause dilated veins on the anterior abdominal wall
d) Usually requires treatment with a venacaval filter
e) Is associated with elevated protein C causing a thrombophilia

[Best Answer = c]

Explanation

Malignancy is often associated with generalised hypercoagulability and DVT. Direct involvement of the vein is relatively rare, but can occur. Another term for hypercoagulability is thrombophilia, which can also be due to specific haematological abnormalities such as protein C deficiency. Iliac vein thrombosis is an uncommon cause of varicose veins. It may lead to visible collateral veins on the anterior abdominal wall. If there is pulmonary embolism despite anticoagulation then a filter may need to be inserted into the inferior vena cava. Filters are not usually used for iliac vein thrombosis alone.

11. Varicose veins

a) If left untreated are a limb threatening condition
b) Always require surgical management
c) Can cause swelling of the whole lower leg
d) If untreated will lead to leg ulceration in many patients
e) Are characterised by loss of competence of the venous valves

[Best Answer = e]

Explanation

> Varicose veins are very common and can usually be managed conservatively unless there are significant skin changes or severe symptoms. In a minority of patients they cause skin changes (varicose eczema or lipodermatosclerosis), which, in some leads ultimately to a venous leg ulcer. If swelling occurs it is usually mild and only affects the ankle. They are associated with incompetence of the venous valves (i.e. the valves do not work to maintain venous blood flow in the correct direction resulting in venous hypertension in the leg).

12. Diabetic feet

a) Are not at risk of gangrene if all pulses are palpable
b) Typically have a proximal pattern of vascular occlusive disease
c) Are resistant to local infection
d) Can be given an all clear if they have a normal ABI
e) Are further compromised due to their loss of sensation

[Best Answer = e]

Explanation

> Diabetics are 50 times more likely to develop gangrene than their non-diabetic counterparts. This is due to a typical distal pattern of vascular occlusive disease affecting the smaller vessels most of all. Gangrene can develop even with palpable pulses. It is further compounded by neuropathy, which results in reduced sensation in the feet. Compromised leucocyte bacterial activity secondary to hyperglycaemia results in more rapid progression of local infection. Paradoxically, due to calcification in arterial walls and microvascular disease, diabetics can be prone to severe tissue loss despite a normal ABI.

13. Deep venous thrombosis

a) Is more common in patients undergoing lower limb surgery
b) Is associated with reduced D-dimer levels
c) Can be prevented by pre-operative warfarinisation of the patient

d) Always results in a swollen painful lower limb
e) All patients should be screened for thrombophilia

[Best Answer = a]

Explanation

> There is a higher incidence of DVT in lower limb surgery due to the subsequent immobility as well as the local trauma. Patients with malignancy are also at much higher risk due to their hypercoaguable state. In DVT D-dimers are usually raised. Preventing DVT pre-operatively is usually a combination of calf compression with stockings and low molecular weight heparinisation. A large percentage of DVTs go unrecognised, particularly when limited to the calf veins, due to lack of symptoms. The majority of pulmonary emboli are from asymptomatic DVTs. Only patients who suffer from an unprovoked DVT (i.e. in the absence of an obvious precipitant) or present with recurrent DVTs or PEs need to be screened for thrombophilia.

14. Popliteal aneurysms

a) Often rupture causing torrential haemorrhage
b) Are rarely bilateral
c) Are associated with aortic aneurysmal disease in > 75% of cases
d) Most commonly present with acute lower limb ischaemia
e) Should be repaired as early as possible to prevent limb loss

[Best Answer = d]

Explanation

> Popliteal aneurysms are commonly bilateral in 50%–70% of patients. Forty to fifty per cent of patients have an abdominal aortic aneurysm. They usually present with acute lower limb ischaemia secondary to thrombosis of the aneurysm or distal embolisation from it. Rupture is extremely rare. Surgical intervention is reserved for those aneurysms greater than 3 cm or those with lots of thrombus, with the remainder being observed with serial ultrasound scans.

15. Lymphoedema

a) Is commonly familial
b) In the world is most frequently caused by malignant infiltration
c) Can be caused by a trivial insect bite
d) Is best treated with aggressive diuretic therapy
e) Responds well to surgical management

[Best Answer = c]

Explanation

In the world the most common cause of lymphoedema is parasitic infestation. In the Western world one of the more common causes is malignant infiltration. True familial lymphoedema (Praecox) is rare. It is normally multi-factorial in origin with even trivial injuries such as an insect bite or minor trauma setting off symptoms and signs. Both surgery and diuretics have very poor long-term results and the principal managements are symptomatic and short-lived.

Case Studies

Case 1

A 65-year-old man presents with the sudden onset of a cold painful right leg. On examination there are no pulses palpable in that leg. A diagnosis is made of an acutely ischaemic leg.

a) What other symptoms may the patient complain of?
b) On examination what would be the key physical signs?
c) What are the two common causes of acute ischaemia of the leg?
d) How long can a leg be severely ischaemic for and still be salvageable?
e) What are the treatment options?
f) What is the role of thrombolysis?
g) How would an embolectomy be performed?
h) What is a fasciotomy and why is it carried out?

Answers

a) The patient may complain of other sensory symptoms (paraesthesiae = pins and needles or numbness) or motor symptoms (weakness or total paralysis) due to ischaemia affecting nerves and muscles.
b) The key findings would be a pale or mottled appearance of the limb, lack of or very sluggish capillary return, weakness of distal muscles (i.e. unable to move toes), absent or reduced sensation distally and coldness of the foot.
c) The two main causes are embolus (e.g. from atrial fibrillation, recent MI, etc.) or thrombosis of a previously diseased distal artery (often there will then be a previous history of claudication).
d) After three to six hours of severe ischaemia muscle and nerves will be irreversibly damaged. Acute ischaemia is therefore a surgical emergency.
e) Occasionally conservative management may be possible if there is only a minor degree of ischaemia. Usually management will be surgical with an embolectomy (if an embolus) or bypass (if thrombosis).
f) Thrombolysis (usually with tissue Plasminogen Activator — tPA) can only be used with less severe cases where the limb is not

immediately threatened. Unlike coronary thrombolysis the t-PA is given by direct low dose infusion directly into the arteries through a catheter inserted into the femoral artery percutaneously. Treatment may take hours or days.

g) Through an incision in the groin the femoral arteries are exposed. This can be done under local or general anaesthetic. A Fogarty catheter is then passed upstream and downstream to clear out the clot. This catheter is long and thin with a balloon on the end. It is passed with the balloon down and easily goes down or through any fresh embolus present. The balloon is then blown up and as the catheter is pulled back it pulls out any embolic material that is present.

h) After reperfusion of an acutely ischaemic leg swelling of the calf muscles will occur. As the muscles swell pressure beneath the fascia of the calf rises and can actually rise to systolic pressure causing secondary ischaemia of these muscles. To prevent this a fasciotomy may be done which is simply an operation to divide the fascia longitudinally to allow the muscles to swell freely.

Case 2

A 73-year-old man presents acutely with abdominal pain radiating into his back and hypotension. On examination there is a pulsatile mass palpable in his abdomen.

a) What is the most likely diagnosis?
b) How should the patient be managed initially?
c) What investigations should be ordered to confirm the diagnosis?
d) What is the expected prognosis of the condition?
e) What are the principles of the surgery?
f) What are the main complications of the operation?

Answers

a) The most likely diagnosis is of a ruptured abdominal aortic aneurysm. Other conditions such as perforated duodenal ulcer or acute pancreatitis can present in a similar way but would not be associated with a pulsatile mass.

b) Once the diagnosis of ruptured aneurysm is suspected the vascular surgeons and duty anaesthetists should be immediately informed. Resuscitation should be started. I.V. access should be sited and blood sent for urgent cross-match (eight units). Blood should also be sent for FBC, U&E's and clotting. If there is time a 12-lead ECG should be performed.

c) No investigations are usually carried out to confirm the diagnosis of ruptured aneurysm, which is made on clinical grounds. Delay may result in the aneurysm rupturing completely and nothing should be allowed to delay getting the patient to theatre.

d) Ruptured aneurysm has an overall mortality rate of 80%–90%. Of the patients who make it to hospital and undergo surgery the mortality rate is approximately 50%.

e) The principle of the operation is to identify and clamp the aorta above and the iliac arteries below the aneurysm. This controls the bleeding. The aneurysm is then opened and an artificial graft is sutured into place to repair the affected section of the aorta. The clamps can then be removed and any remaining bleeding points can then be dealt with. The aneurysm sac is then sutured over the graft and the abdomen is closed.

f) The main complications are uncontrollable bleeding leading to death on the table, myocardial infarction and post-operative respiratory and renal failure.

Case 3

A 65-year-old man presents with a history of several episodes of loss of vision in the left eye lasting less than five minutes each.

a) What symptom is he describing?
b) What investigations should be performed?
c) What drug therapies should be started?
d) What are the indications for surgery?
e) Which operation is usually performed for this condition?
f) What are the risks of surgery?

Answers

a) Amaurosis fugax. This is transient blindness affecting one eye only. It is due to an embolus passing though the retinal circulation. It is often described as "like a curtain coming across the vision".

b) After a full history and examination and routine blood tests a Duplex scan of the carotid arteries should be ordered to see if there is a significant stenosis of the internal carotid artery.

c) All patients with TIA's should be started on an antiplatelet agent such as aspirin or clopidogrel. They should also be started on a lipid lowering agent (usually a statin) and appropriate antihypertensives, usually with an ACE inhibitor.

d) Carotid endarterectomy is indicated for symptomatic disease (prior stroke, TIA or amaurosis) in patients with an internal carotid artery stenosis greater than 70%.

e) The usual operation is carotid endarterectomy. Some centres are now using carotid stenting in selected cases.

f) The main risk of carotid endarterectomy is the risk of causing a stroke. This risk should be less than 5% in the hands of an experienced vascular surgeon. Other risks include damage to cranial nerves, particularly the Vagus (causing hoarseness of the voice by interruption of recurrent laryngeal nerve fibres) and the hypoglossal nerve (causes the tongue to deviate to the side of the lesion).

Case 4

A young man with no previous medical history was involved in a motorcycle crash with a deforming injury to his left thigh. This is his only injury. On arrival to the hospital his left leg is shortened and abducted and flexed with a swollen upper thigh. He is hypotensive with a BP of 90/55. He has lost sensation in his foot, which looks dusky and mottled with no evidence of movement in the toes.

a) What is the cause of his left leg symptoms?
b) Why is he hypotensive?
c) What complication has he sustained as a result of the injury?
d) What is the initial management of this patient?

e) If his leg fails to improve with initial measures what investigations should be carried out?

Answers

a) He has sustained a fracture to the shaft of his left femur. This is indicated by the shortening and abduction and is a common injury sustained in motorcycle crashes.
b) Fractures of the femur can result in blood loss of up to two litres which could explain his hypotension. It would be important to exclude other causes of hypotension by excluding haemorrhage in other parts of the body.
c) He has sustained a vascular injury probably to the superficial femoral artery due to either direct crushing trauma or secondary to the fracture with the vessel either being "nipped" or transacted by the jagged bony ends.
d) Initial management must be ABCDE as per ATLS guidelines. As far as the leg is concerned the application of a splint (Thomas) not only reduces pain but could also spontaneously correct the vascular injury by re-aligning the fractured femur which might restore flow in the artery.
e) The gold standard would be an angiogram after consulting a vascular surgeon. This enables the vessel injury to be mapped and surgery to be planned accordingly.

Case 5

A 79-year-old woman is admitted two weeks following a total knee replacement. She takes tamoxifen. She complains of breathlessness at rest with some pain on deep inspiration and a cough with some blood in her sputum.

a) What is the most likely diagnosis?
b) What risk factors does she have for this condition?
c) What investigations can be carried out?
d) What is the management of her condition?
e) What preventative measures can be taken against her condition?
f) She has a daughter who is about to undergo an arthroscopy. She asks if he condition is a familial one?

Answers

a) The most likely diagnosis is a pulmonary embolus.

b) Her risk factors are age, surgery (particularly lower limb surgery), immobility post-op. and malignancy (tamoxifen for breast cancer).

c) A good history and examination will reveal the diagnosis. Other confirmatory tests include: CXR, ECG, arterial blood gases, V/Q scan and more commonly today, CT pulmonary angiogram. Very rarely pulmonary arteriography can be carried out.

d) Resuscitate and provide supplemental oxygen and analagesia. Immediate heparinisation with either intravenous heparin or low molecular weight heparin. Occasionally patients can have thrombolysis but not following recent surgery. Pulmonary embolectomy is rarely available.

e) Stop the pill or HRT. TED stockings, subcutaneous heparin, early mobilisation and mechanical calf compression.

f) Venous thrombo-embolism can be hereditary in patients with forms of thrombophilia. However these diseases present with unprovoked events and it is unlikely that this lady's event was related to thrombophilia.

Extended Matching Questions

EMQ 1

a. Diabetes
b. Buerger's disease
c. Vasculitis
d. Atherosclerosis
e. Syphilis
f. Marfan's syndrome
g. Tuberculosis
h. Takayasu's disease
i. Popliteal aneurysm
j. Thrombophilia

Choose the diagnosis from the list above, which most fits the case scenarios described below:

1) A 24-year-old man presents with a gangrenous toe. His only known risk factor is smoking.
2) A 60-year-old man presents with emboli to the toes of his right leg. He has had a previous abdominal aortic aneurysm repair. Peripheral pulses are easily palpable.
3) A 39-year-old lady presents with a DVT. She has previously been treated for an embolus to her right arm. She is otherwise well and has no vascular risk factors.
4) A 50-year-old man presents with an abdominal aneurysm. There is a family history of his father and uncle also having aneurysms.
5) A 28-year-old lady presents with dizziness and blurred vision on sitting up and on examination has absent pulses in both arms. She is a non-smoker.

Answers

> **1) b.**
> Buerger's disease, also known as thromboangiitis obliterans, is an inflammatory arteritis affecting the smaller arteries, found only in young male smokers. It is rare in the UK but common in Asia and the Far East.

2) i.

Popliteal aneurysms are commonly found in patients with abdominal aneurysms. Rupture is rare and distal embolisation or thrombosis are more common complications.

3) j.

Thrombophilia is a tendency to form blood clots due to a haematological abnormality such as a deficiency of protein C, protein S, or antithrombin. These factors are screened for by asking the haematology lab for a "thrombophilia screen".

4) d.

Abdominal aneurysms often run in families but are usually still atherosclerotic in origin.

5) h.

Takayasu's is a rare inflammatory arteritis more common in countries such as Japan. It affects the upper limb and carotid arteries of young women.

EMQ 2

a. Amputation
b. Aneurysm stenting (endovascular repair)
c. Urgent CT scan of abdomen
d. Ultrasound scan of abdomen
e. Referral for anaesthetic assessment
f. Emergency aneurysm repair
g. Conservative management
h. Elective aneurysm repair
i. Work up for lower limb bypass graft
j. Ultrasound of popliteal arteries

Select the most appropriate option for the patients described below:

1) A 65-year-old smoker with COPD and angina is found to have a 6.5 cm infrarenal aortic aneurysm on routine ultrasound scanning.
2) A 50-year-old man is referred from the orthopaedic clinic because of the finding of a pulsatile mass behind the left knee.
3) An otherwise fit 65-year-old man is found to have an asymptomatic abdominal aneurysm on clinical examination.

4) A 70-year-old man is admitted with acute onset abdominal and back pain, a pulsatile mass and a systolic pressure of 75 mmHg.

5) An 85-year-old man with known metastatic lung cancer is admitted with acute onset abdominal and back pain. His blood pressure is 70 systolic, his Glasgow Coma Score is 8 and his creatinine is 425 μmol/L.

Answers

1) e.
Aneurysms greater than 5.5 cm should be repaired if the patient is fit enough. This patient needs an anaesthetic opinion before going ahead with surgery.

2) j.
This is likely to be a popliteal aneurysm.

3) d.
He should have an ultrasound to assess the size of the aneurysm.

4) f.
This is a ruptured aneurysm and needs immediate urgent surgery. There is no time for investigations such as CT scanning.

5) g.
This is also likely to be a ruptured aneurysm but with the co-morbidities described the patient could not possibly survive surgery and conservative (palliative) treatment is indicated.

EMQ 3

a. Compression stockings
b. Venal caval filter
c. Thrombophilia screen
d. Amputation
e. Skin grafting
f. Compression bandaging
g. Sapheno-popliteal ligation
h. Biopsy
i. Angiogram or duplex scan
j. Endovascular surgery

Select the most appropriate treatment option or investigation for the patients described below:

1) A 56-year-old man with long saphenous varicose veins and no symptoms or skin changes.
2) A 65-year-old lady with breast cancer who is on long term warfarin and has a large pulmonary embolism.
3) A 70-year-old lady with lipodermatosclerosis and a leg ulcer.
4) A 65-year-old man with pain in his foot at night, absent foot pulses and a large ulcer on his foot.
5) A 70-year-old lady with normal pulses and a leg ulcer which is failing to heal despite compression bandaging.

Answers

1) a.
Asymptomatic uncomplicated veins can be managed conservatively with compression stockings.

2) b.
Pulmonary embolus despite adequate anticoagulation is an indication for an IVC filter.

3) f.
Lipodermatosclerois results from chronic venous disease. Venous leg ulcers should be treated with compression bandages if the ABI excludes significant arterial disease.

4) i.
This patient probably has critical ischaemia. ABI could be measured to help confirm this. Angiogram or Duplex will show if they are suitable for an angioplasty or bypass.

5) h.
A chronic non-healing leg ulcer may have undergone malignant change (Marjolin's ulcer) and should be biopsied.

EMQ 4

a. A beta-blocker
b. Aspirin and dipyridamole

c. A statin
d. Low molecular weight heparin subcutaneously
e. Heparin infusion intravenously
f. Antibiotics
g. Gabapentin
h. Atenolol
i. Gabapentinj
j. Digoxin

Select the most appropriate treatment option for the patients described below:

1) A 58-year-old man presents to the clinic with pain on walking in his left calf after 200 metres. He has no pain at rest and manages to be self-caring.
2) A 68-year-old woman who has recently had an amputation complains of pain and redness in the stump.
3) A 70-year-old man with a past history of claudication at 150 yards now presents as an emergency with sudden onset of pain and loss of sensation and power in the affected leg.
4) A 61-year-old woman is admitted for a fem-pop bypass graft tomorrow. She is otherwise fit and well.
5) A 33-year-old girl presents with her second DVT out of the blue. Her mother died suddenly aged 40.

Answers

1) c.
This patient is likely to have intermittent claudication. If confirmed he should be started on treatment to reduce vascular risk factors including aspirin and a statin. Aspirin and dipyridamole is uaually reserved for patients after stroke or TIA.

2) f.
She probably has a stump infection. Another possibility, especially if swelling is prominent, is a DVT in the stump.

3) e.
This patient has acute ischaemia. Heparin should be started immediately to prevent further thrombosis or embolisation, most will also need emergency surgery.

4) d.

Subcutaneous, prophylactic heparin is started to prevent perioperative DVT.

5) e.

She probably has a thrombophilia. With two events she should be initially heparinised and then subsequently converted to warfarin.

EMQ 5

a. Buttock pain on walking
b. Pain in the calf at night
c. Gangrene of the big toe
d. Transient ischaemic attacks affecting the left arm
e. Pigmentation on medial side of calf
f. Pain in back
g. Dizziness on standing
h. Weakness of legs
i. Pain in the calf on walking
j. Transient blindness affecting the left eye

Suggest the most likely symptom for the patients types described below:

1) A patient with critical ischaemia.
2) A significant left internal carotid stenosis.
3) A patient with a large but not ruptured abdominal aneurysm.
4) A patient with deep venous insufficiency.
5) A patient with an acute femoral embolus.

Answers

1) c.

Critical ischaemia is manifested by vascular rest pain felt in the toes or foot, worse at night. It may lead to ulceration or gangrene.

2) j.

Transient blindness (= amaurosis fujax) is a form of transient ischaemic attack. It affects the ipsilateral (same side) eye as the internal carotid stenosis.

3) f.

Aneurysms may cause back or abdominal pain.

4) e.

Deep venous insufficiency causes pigmentation and lipodermato-sclerosis, normally on the medial side of the calf. It may lead on to a leg ulcer.

5) h.

Acute ischaemia causes the 6 "P's" — pain, pallor, paraesthesiae, pulseless, paralysis and perishing cold! Paralysis (muscle ischaemia) results in weakness of the affected leg.

Chapter 11   Urology

Roy McGregor

Roy McGregor

Multiple Choice Questions

[Each single best answer (SBA) question comprises a stem and a number of answers. You are asked to decide which single item represents the best answer to the question.]

1. Catheterisation

a) Acute urinary retention is an uncommon urological indication for catheterisation
b) Foley catheters are retained in the bladder by a coiling device
c) Is performed using a clean technique
d) Suprapubic catheters (SPC) are used instead of urethral catheters in patients presenting with frank haematuria and clot retention
e) Urethral stricture is a recognised complication

[Best Answer = e]

Explanation

Acute urinary retention is a common urological indication for catheterisation. Foley catheters are retained in the bladder by a balloon located at the tip of the catheter, which is inflated with sterile water. Catheterisation should be performed using an aseptic technique in order to avoid inserting bacteria into the urinary tract. SPC's should be avoided in patients suspected of having bladder cancer (i.e. presenting with haematuria) because of the risk of seeding along the catheter tract. SPC's are used when urethral catheterisation is not possible due to blockage (e.g. benign prostatic hypertrophy (BPH), prostate cancer, urethral stricture, etc.) or disruption of the urethra or when long-term catheterisation is required. To prevent urethral trauma do not forget the golden rule of catheterisation — never blow up the balloon until you have seen the golden flow of urine! Complications of urethral catheterisation include infection, bleeding, urethral trauma and strictures.

2. Painless frank haematuria

a) Indicates cancer of the urinary tract until proven otherwise
b) Is usually caused by kidney stones
c) Is often mimicked by ranitidine
d) A computerised tomography (CT) scan of the abdomen is mandatory
e) Usually indicates an infection of the urinary tract

[Best Answer = a]

Explanation

> Painless frank haematuria should be presumed cancerous until proven otherwise. Approximately 35% of patients have a bladder or renal cell carcinoma. Whilst kidney stones can cause painless frank haematuria, it is much more common for them to present with painful haematuria, especially as the stone passes into the ureter blocking the flow of urine resulting in renal (ureteric) colic. Rifampicin may colour the urine orange/red, ranitidine does not. An abdominal CT scan is usually only performed if a renal tumour is suspected on ultrasound scan (USS) or intravenous urogram (IVU). When associated with a urinary tract infection frank haemarturia is usually accompanied with pain (dysuria).

3. Which of the following statements about benign prostatic hyperplasia (BPH) is false?

a) Arises from the peripheral zone of the prostate
b) Is generally a disease of elderly men
c) Trans-urethral resection of the prostate (TURP) is the most common surgical treatment
d) Is commonly treated with alpha-blockers
e) Can lead to renal failure

[Best Answer = a]

Explanation

> BPH usually arises from the transitional zone unlike cancer, which usually arises in the peripheral zone. The incidence of benign prostatic

hypertrophy increases with age. Alpha-blockers relax the muscle within the prostate and around the bladder neck, decreasing bladder out flow obstruction (BOO). TURP is still the most common surgical treatment, however many patients are treated medically. BPH results in BOO and lower urinary tract symptoms (LUTS). Severe BOO can result in renal dilation (hydronephrosis) and renal failure (obstructive nephropathy).

4. **Voiding (obstructive) urinary symptoms include**

   a) Frequency
   b) Haematuria
   c) Hesitancy
   d) Urgency
   e) Nocturia

[Best Answer = c]

Explanation

Lower urinary tract symptoms (LUTS) are classified as voiding (previously known as obstructive) or storage (previously known as irritative) symptoms. Haematuria is a sign not a symptom and is not usually associated with BOO. Voiding symptoms are usually related to BOO and include hesitancy and straining to commence micturition, passage of a weak intermittent stream, terminal dribbling and a sensation of incomplete emptying. Occasionally voiding symptoms are due to bladder muscle failure. Storage symptoms can be due to BOO but may be due to other intravesical causes including urinary tract infection (UTI), bladder stones and bladder cancer. Storage symptoms consist of frequency, nocturia (need to wake from sleep more than once during the night to pee), urgency and urge incontinence.

5. **Prostate cancer**

   a) Is the most common cancer in men in the Western world
   b) Incidence is decreasing
   c) Elevated serum prostate specific antigen (PSA) indicates the presence of prostate cancer

d) Can be treated with testosterone

e) Always requires intervention

[Best Answer = a]

Explanation

In the Western world prostate cancer is the most common cancer in men. The incidence has been increasing partly due to an increased use of serum PSA to detect prostate cancer. Whilst an elevated PSA can be due to cancer, it can also be raised due to infection of the prostate; instrumentation of the urethra; or a very large gland (BPH). It is very sensitive at detecting something wrong with the prostate gland but not very specific for prostate cancer. Treatment options are many and depend on the life expectancy of the patient, the stage and grade of the cancer, the patient's choice and the services available. Prostate cancer growth is stimulated by testosterone, therefore, reducing circulating testosterone levels by surgical or pharmacological castration is a treatment option. Asymptomatic elderly patients with a life expectancy of less than ten years are often put on a watchful waiting programme, the aim being palliation if and when symptoms arise.

6. **Ureteric (Renal) colic**

a) Colic from a lower third ureteric stone can be referred to the buttocks

b) Usually requires surgical intervention

c) Is associated with (micro or macro) haematuria in approximately 90% of cases

d) Is best investigated by an IVU

e) The size of the stone correlates with severity of the pain

[Best Answer = c]

Explanation

Blockage of the ureter usually results in severe colicky pain that radiates from the loin around to the groin. This may continue into the scrotum or labia majora if the stone is in the lower third of the ureter. The majority of stones are < 4 mm and have a 90% chance of passing therefore do not require surgical intervention. Trauma to the urothelium by a stone causes micro and/or macroscopic haematuria in over 90% of cases. The non-contrast CT scan has taken over from IVU as being the investigation of choice for renal colic. The size of the stone does not correlate with the severity of the pain.

7. Testicular torsion

a) Occurs most frequently between the ages of two and ten years
b) The underlying cause is known as the "ball and chain" abnormality
c) Is commonly associated with dysuria
d) Classically it presents as a painful, high riding testicle with a horizontal lie
e) Can be treated expectantly to see if they untwist

[Best Answer = d]

Explanation

Testicular torsion can occur at any age but commonly occurs between the ages of 12 to 27 years. It is associated with an underlying congenital abnormality known as the "bell-clapper" deformity where the tunica vaginalis has a high attachment to the spermatic cord and not the testicle, like a bell-clapper. This allows the testicle to twist on the cord resulting in its blood supply being cut off. Classically they present having had a sudden onset of testicular pain, and no other lower urinary tract symptoms. On examination the testicle is exquisitely painful often preventing examination, high in the scrotum with a horizontal lie. Suspected cases are a urological emergency and require immediate surgical exploration otherwise the testicle may die and require removal.

8. Bladder cancer

a) Is related to drinking coffee
b) In the UK > 90% are transitional cell carcinomas (TCC's)

c) Affects ten times as many men as women

d) Commonly present as recurrent urinary tract infections

e) Usually requires surgery to remove the bladder

[Best Answer = b]

Explanation

> Bladder cancer is not related to coffee consumption; 51% of male and 31% of female bladder TCC's are related to cigarette smoking; 98% of tumours in the UK are transitional cell carcinomas, with squamous cell carcinomas and adenocarcinomas making up the other 2%. The male to female ratio is 3:1, although this is levelling out as more women take up smoking. Bladder cancers usually present with pain-less haematuria, however 15% present as recurrent UTI's; 85% of bladder cancers are superficial and are treated by endoscopic resec-tion and/or intravesical chemo and/or immunotherapy. A radical cys-tectomy is typically done for fit patients with aggressive and/or muscle invasive disease. Patients unfit for surgery can be treated with radiotherapy.

9. Suprapubic catheters (SPC's)

a) Should be inserted when the bladder is empty

b) Are inserted 2 cm below the umbilicus

c) Is the first choice of catheter for patients in acute urinary retention

d) Complications include bowel perforation

e) Should always be inserted in theatre under aseptic conditions

[Best Answer = d]

Explanation

> The anterior wall of a full bladder is in contact with the anterior abdominal wall but an empty bladder has intervening loops of bowel, which are at risk of perforation. The first choice of catheter used for patients in acute urinary retention is a Foley catheter as it is less

invasive. In spite of these precautions bowel perforations can occur. SPC's are inserted above the pubic symphysis in the midline under aseptic conditions. This is often done in A&E.

10. Testicular tumours

a) Seminomas are the most aggressive and rapid growing tumours
b) Make up 2% of male malignancies
c) A radical orchidectomy is performed through a scrotal incision
d) A testicular lump should be investigated if it changes in size, shape or consistency
e) Carcinoembryonic antigen (CEA) is a tumour marker for some testicular tumours

[Best Answer = b]

Explanation

Seminomas grow slowly unlike other types of testicular cancers. Testicular tumours make up 2% of all male malignancies. A radical orchidectomy is performed through an inguinal incision so the spermatic cord can be clamped before manipulation of the tumour preventing dissemination of cancer cells. It also allows the testicular cord to be taken with testicle. Suspicious testicular lumps should always be investigated with an urgent ultrasound scan. Alpha-feto protein, beta-human chorionic gonadotrophin and placental alkaline phosphatase are produced by some testicular tumours.

11. Renal cell carcinoma (RCC)

a) Accounts for 80% of malignant renal tumours
b) An USS is always diagnostic
c) Often present as a right sided varicocoele
d) Are related to smoking
e) Over 80% of patients present with loin pain

[Best Answer = a]

Explanation

> RCC is the most common malignant tumour of the kidney accounting for 80% of all malignant renal tumours. Benign simple cysts are the most common renal mass. Although an USS can detect a renal mass, a contrast CT scan is typically required to make the diagnosis. The left testicular vein drains into the left renal vein, whereas the right testicular vein drains into the inferior vena cava. Consequently, if a tumour grows into the left renal vein it can obstruct the left testicular vein causing a varicocoele. Patients presenting with a left sided varicocoele should have an ultrasound scan of their left kidney. RCC's are not related to smoking; 50% of RCC's present as an asymptomatic incidental finding on ultrasound or CT scan.

12. Kidney stones

a) Ninety per cent of kidney stones are radio-opaque.
b) Urate stones are best visualised by an IVP
c) Kidney stones tend to get stuck in the mid ureter
d) Stones 1 cm or less will usually pass spontaneously
e) Percutaneous nephrolithotomy (PCNL) is usually performed to remove stones in the ureter

[Best Answer = a]

Explanation

> Ninety per cent of kidney stones have calcium in them, which renders them radiopaque (unlike gallstones, of which 90% are radiolucent). Urate stones however are radiolucent and are best visualised by a non-contrast CT scan. Stones tend to get stuck at one of three narrowings in the ureter; the pelvic ureteric junction (PUJ), where the ureter crosses the pelvic brim over the iliac vessels and the vesico-ureteric junction (VUJ). Stones 5 mm or less have a 95% chance of passing spontaneously in three weeks and so are left to pass of there own accord provided the pain can be controlled with oral analgesia and they do not develop complications such as an infection. PCNL is performed to remove large stones in the kidney that are too big for extra-corporeal shock wave lithotripsy (ESWL).

13. Routine investigations for haematuria do not include

a) Urea and electrolytes
b) Ultrasound scan of kidneys, ureters and bladder (KUB)
c) Full blood count
d) Angiogram
e) Flexible cystoscopy

[Best Answer = d]

Explanation

All patients presenting with microscopic or macroscopic haematuria of unknown origin should have a set of investigations, a "haematuria screen", to determine the cause. Urine is sent for culture and sensitivity to rule out an infection and for cytological evaluation to look for cancerous cells. Blood should be sent for a full blood count to determine if the patient is anaemic, has an infection or low platelets. Clotting studies should also be performed as well as urea and creatinine to determine renal function. If the patient is a man over 45 years some centres will perform a serum PSA to rule out prostate cancer. A KUB ultrasound scan and X-ray are easy and cheap ways of detecting renal and bladder lesions. Patients should also have an IVP to rule out TCC's in the upper tracts. Angiograms are rarely performed. A flexible or rigid cystoscopy is performed to directly visualise the bladder mucosa.

14. Which of the following is not a complication of bladder outflow obstruction (BOO)?

a) Interstitial cystitis
b) Bladder calculi
c) Acute urinary retention (AUR)
d) Obstructive nephropathy
e) Urinary tract infections (UTI)

[Best Answer = a]

Explanation

> Interstitial cystitis is an idiopathic chronic painful inflammatory process of the bladder, which is not related to BOO. BOO can result in the bladder failing to contract strongly enough to expel all the urine. This can result in a significant volume of urine being left in the bladder after each void. This residual volume of stagnant urine acts as a breeding ground for bacteria resulting in UTI's both of which pre-dispose to bladder calculi formation. In severe cases the patient is unable to urinate at all and develops AUR. In severe cases of BOO patients can develop chronic retention of urine such that the bladder is permanently full which prevents adequate drainage of the kidneys. This "back up" of pressure reduces the kidneys' ability to filter urine, resulting in renal impairment, known as obstructive nephropathy.

15. Testicular cancer

a) Is usually painful
b) Often spreads to the inguinal lymph nodes
c) Supraclavicular lymph nodes need to be examined
d) Typically transilluminate
e) All produce androgens

[Best Answer = c]

Explanation

> Ten per cent of malignant tumours are painful. Lymph node drainage does not include the inguinal nodes but does include the abdominal, supraclavicular and mediastinal lymph nodes. Malignancies tend to be solid and do not transilluminate. Sertoli cell tumours can produce oestrogens and androgens, which results in feminisation and swelling of the breast tissue (gynaecomastia) or virilisation.

Case Studies

Case 1

A fit 65-year-old man presents with a six-month history of hesitancy, straining and a weak urinary stream. On digital rectal examination he is found to have a non-tender hard irregular prostate.

a) What is the most likely diagnosis?
b) What test would you perform to confirm the diagnosis?
c) Based on the digital rectal examination, what T stage would it be?
d) What investigations would you request to stage the disease?
e) He is found to have localised disease and wants surgery — what treatment options are open to him?
f) What are the complications associated with surgical intervention?
g) What other treatment options are there for him?
h) After treatment how are these patients followed up?

Answers

a) Prostate cancer is the most likely diagnosis. Prostatic calcification can also feel hard on digital rectal examination but in this age group it should be considered as cancerous until proven otherwise.

b) An abnormal rectal examination or an elevated prostate specific antigen level is enough to prompt a prostate biopsy. Prostate tissue is required to make a histological diagnosis. Occasionally if the patient is very unwell and has overt prostate cancer on rectal examination with a very high PSA or a positive bone scan, a biopsy is not required to make the diagnosis. Prostate biopsies are usually performed in the day surgery unit or the outpatient department and involve the use of a trans-rectal ultrasound (TRUS) probe to visualise the prostate and a tru-cut biopsy needle to take systematic biopsies.

c) T2. Prostate cancer is staged using the tumour nodes metastases (TNM) classification, T stage as follows:

T0 — No tumour identified
T1 — None palpable
T2 — Palpable but confined to the prostate

T3 — Palpable with extra-capsular spread

T4 — Locally invading or fixed to pelvic sidewall

d) Staging of prostate cancer involves a blood test for PSA, which is a prostate cancer tumour marker. PSA levels vary according to the size of the gland, the presence of infection and the presence and extent of prostate cancer. If the PSA is very high metastatic disease should be suspected and a bone scan or CT or MRI scan of the abdomen and pelvis performed. Prostate cancer usually metastasises to bone resulting in osteoblastic lesions, which can be seen on a bone scan. Lymph node metastases or capsular breaches are best seen on a CT or MRI scan.

e) Assuming he is in good health, with a life expectancy of greater than ten years, the intent of treatment would be curative. Current surgical options include a radical prostatectomy. This can be performed as an open or laparoscopic procedure. Recently robotic surgery has also been employed.

f) Regardless of the surgical technique used a significant number of patients suffer from incontinence and impotence. Remember complications can be classified as immediate, early or late and are either related to the anaesthetic or surgery.

g) Other curative treatment options include external beam radiotherapy, the implantation of radioactive seeds or wires (brachytherapy). Experimental work using high intensity focused ultrasound (HIFU) and cryotherapy is underway.

h) After curative treatment, regardless of the modality, patients are reviewed on a regular basis in clinic to check that they are not developing a recurrence or complications. This involves a targeted history and examination (including a digital rectal examination) to detect localised recurrence (lower urinary tract symptoms), bone metastases (back pain/neurological symptoms) and generalised symptoms of recurrent metastatic disease (weight loss and lethargy). Investigations include PSA, LFT's and U&E's. If any of the above is abnormal further investigations should be performed.

Case 2

A fit 72-year-old man presents with his first episode of acute urinary retention. During the previous week he was having increased difficulty in passing urine.

Coincidentally he had also developed sinusitis for which he was taking systemic nasal decongestants and painkillers that had made him constipated. On catheterisation he drained 800 ml of urine and digital rectal examination revealed an enlarged benign feeling prostate.

a) What part of the prostate gland does benign prostatic hyperplasia commonly arise?

b) What symptoms might he have had during the previous week?

c) Name some of the precipitating factors for acute urinary retention?

d) Is acute urinary retention always painful?

e) What investigations would you do?

f) What is the initial management?

g) He goes into retention again later that year in spite of being on maximum medical treatment. What treatment options are available?

h) He decides that he wants to have a trans-urethral resection of the prostate (TURP). What do you need to warn him about during consenting?

Answers

a) Benign prostatic hyperplasia arises in the transitional zone of the prostate unlike prostate cancer, which arises in the peripheral zone.

b) During the previous week his bladder was probably failing to empty completely because of bladder outflow obstruction caused by the enlarged prostate. He would have developed significant voiding symptoms such as hesitancy, straining with the passage of a weak, intermittent stream and a sensation of incomplete emptying. If the bladder is chronically obstructed it can become "irritable" resulting in storage symptoms such as frequency, urgency and nocturia.

c) Constipation can precipitate acute urinary retention (AUR). Impaired bladder contractility can result from bladder muscle inflammation secondary to a urinary tract infection. Over-distension of the bladder reduces contractility of the bladder muscle (same principle as Starlings Law of the heart). This usually occurs due to social reasons, e.g. stuck in traffic, or a depressed level of consciousness, e.g. excessive alcohol intake. Drugs that have anticholinergic side effects inhibit detrusor muscle contractility, e.g. atropine, tricyclic antidepressants. Pseudoephedrine (an alpha-receptor agonist used as a nasal decongestant) increases the internal sphincter tone of the bladder neck, increasing bladder outflow obstruction. The post-operative period is a common time for patients to go into retention usually as a result of a combination of many factors including pain and constipation caused by opiate analgesia plus spinal anaesthesia and poor mobility.

d) Acute urinary retention is often defined as the painful inability to pass urine and implies a relatively acute onset, while chronic is defined as the painless inability to pass urine and implies a chronic, slowly developing process. Occasionally retention can occur acutely and be painless. This occurs after a spinal anaesthetic or spinal injury. There is also such a thing as acute on chronic retention.

e) *Blood*: FBC (WCC); U&E's (renal impairment).
Urine: Urinalysis; microscopy, culture and sensitivity (MC&S).
Radiology: Ultrasound scan of the kidneys, ureters and bladder (if renal impairment is present).

f) After catheterisation one should correct or remove any precipitating factors. Start the patient on an alpha-blocker to relax the smooth muscle around the bladder neck and in the prostate, reducing bladder outflow obstruction. The catheter is then removed to see if the patient can void. He could also be started on finasteride, a 5-alpha reductase inhibitor that stops the conversion of testosterone to the more active ingredient dihydrotestosterone in the prostate resulting in shrinkage of the prostate gland. Often patients are given lifestyle advice to reduce the bother from lower urinary tract symptoms such as decreasing intake of caffeine, alcohol and fluids.

g) As he was on maximum medical treatment and this was his second episode of retention the likelihood of it happening again is very high. Consequently he should be offered definitive treatment. The current gold standard remains TURP although many newer techniques are being used (e.g. laser enucleation or vapourization).

h) The patient should be told about the small possibility of detecting cancer, the operation and its various complications. Complications are split into early and late. Early complications include TUR syndrome (dilutional hyponatraemia secondary to absorption of the hypotonic irrigant), lower urinary tract infections including sepsis and septic shock, epididymo-orchitis and blood loss requiring a blood transfusion. Late complications include retrograde ejaculation (75%); erectile dysfunction (5%); incontinence; urethral stricture; and re-growth of the prostate. General risks including DVT and pulmonary embolism as well as anaesthetic risks should also be mentioned.

Case 3

A 34-year-old man presents with rigours and severe colicky right-sided loin to groin pain. He is flushed, hot and sweaty. On examination he has a temperature of 38°C, pulse of 110 bpm and is mildly hypotensive. Several years earlier he had required surgery to remove a left ureteric stone.

a) What is the most likely diagnosis?
b) What complication has he developed?
c) What radiological investigation(s) is/are required to confirm the diagnosis?
d) What other investigations are required?
e) Which organisms are commonly associated with struvite stones?
f) What is the immediate treatment?

Answers

a) The most likely diagnosis is right ureteric colic with an associated infected obstructed kidney. People having had one episode of ureteric colic have a greater chance of another episode.

b) He has developed severe sepsis and is probably in the early stages of septic shock.

c) He requires an IVU or non-contrast CT scan or renal USS and KUB X-ray. The old gold standard was an IVU. Recently non-contrast spiral CT scan of the abdomen and pelvis has been shown to be more sensitive and specific than an IVU.

d) *Blood*: FBC, U&E's, clotting, culture and sensitivity.
    Urine: Urinalysis, MC&S.

e) Proteus, Pseudomonas, Klebsiella.

f) Immediate treatment includes IV fluid resuscitation, IV antibiotics, nursing in a high dependency unit with close monitoring of fluid balance. An urgent nephrostomy tube needs to be inserted into the kidney to drain the infected urine.

Case 4

A 24-year-old man presents with a 2 × 2 × 2 cm painless testicular mass. It has doubled in size over the last three months. On examination one can get above it and it is intratesticular. The cord had a hard lump in it a few centimetres proximal to the testicle.

a) Classify testicular tumours giving frequency of occurrence.
b) List the risk factors for testicular cancers.
c) What is the first radiological investigation that needs to be ordered urgently?
d) Clinically what stage is it?
e) What operation does he need?
f) What are the potential risks of surgery?
g) What are the fundamental principles of this operation?

Answers

a) Only 5% of testicular tumours are benign (cysts, microlithiasis, etc.). Almost all are malignant (95%).
   Testicular tumours can be divided into germ cell and non-germ cell tumours. Almost all are germ cell tumours (> 90%). The germ cell tumours can be divided into seminomas (40%), non-seminomatous germ cell tumours or NSGCT (10%) (also called teratomas) and mixed (40%). Rarely, choriocarcinomas and yolk sac tumours are seen (these are types of NSGCT). Non-germ cell tumours are rare (< 10%) and include Leydig cell and Sertoli cell tumours and lymphomas.
b) Testicular maldescent and testicular agenesis or dysgenesis.
c) Scrotal ultrasound scan.
d) T3, as it is invading the spermatic cord.
e) He needs an urgent radical orchidectomy.
f) The potential risks of surgery are minimal and the procedure is often done as a day case under a general anaesthetic. Risks include haematoma, ilio-inguinal nerve damage, making a hole in the scrotal skin, wound infection, local recurrence and general anaesthetic risk.
g) As this is a cancer operation the fundamental principles are to avoid dissemination of tumour cells into the circulation and preventing spillage of tumour cells locally. This is achieved by making a groin incision through which the cord is isolated and clamped gaining vascular control prior manipulation of the testicle.

The testicle is then delivered through the wound and examined having isolated the wound with swabs. If obviously cancerous it is removed with the cord. An inguinal incision also reduces the risk of accidentally incising the tumour at the time of a scrotal incision and avoiding spillage of tumour cells and possible seeding in the scrotal skin.

Case 5

A 75-year-old heavy smoker presents with a three-week history of intermittent painless frank haematuria. He has been losing weight for several months and had a urinary tract infection six weeks ago.

a) What is the most likely diagnosis?
b) What are the risk factors?
c) A bladder biopsy reveals high grade muscle invasive disease. What T stage would that make it?
d) Staging scans show that it is confined to the bladder. What are the treatment options?
e) What percentage of superficial cancers progress to muscle invasive cancers?
f) What is the most common type of bladder cancer found in the UK?

Answers

a) Bladder cancer.
b) Smoking (nitrosamines), exposure to analine dyes and aromatic amines used in the rubber, printing and leather industries, chronic *Schistosomiasis haematobium* infection, chronic irradiation, long-term catheterisation, cyclophosphamide therapy.
c) T2.
d) The treatment options depend on whether he is fit enough for an operation. If he was he should have his bladder removed (radical cystectomy) and an ileal conduit formed. If he was young and motivated a new bladder (neobladder) could be made from ileum. If he is not fit for surgery he should have radiotherapy.
e) Fifteen per cent.
f) Transitional cell carcinoma.

Extended Matching Questions

EMQ 1

a. Bladder cancer
b. Ureteric (renal) colic
c. Benign prostatic hyperplasia
d. Testicular tumour
e. Prostate cancer
f. UTI
g. Inguino-scrotal hernia
h. Epididymal cyst
i. Urethral stricture
j. Hydrocoele

Choose the diagnosis from the list above, which most fits the case scenarios described below:

1) A 65-year-old male who is a heavy smoker presents with one episode of painless frank haematuria throughout the stream.
2) A 29-year-old man presents with hesitancy, straining and the passage of a weak fine stream with a sensation of incomplete emptying. Several years earlier he had contracted gonorrhoea.
3) A 32-year-old male chef presents to casualty clutching his abdomen rolling around on the floor with severe loin and left-sided colicky abdominal pain, frequency and urgency of urination, nausea and vomiting.
4) A 25-year-recently married lady presents with frequency, urgency, dysuria and the passage of small volumes of urine.
5) A 45-year-old man presents with a painless 5 × 5 × 6 cm right-sided scrotal swelling which has come on slowly over the past nine months. On examination one can get above it. The overlying skin is normal, the testicle cannot be felt separate from the swelling which transilluminates brightly.

Answers

> **1) a.**
> The incidence of bladder cancer increases with age and is more common in men than women. Smoking is a risk factor. Bladder cancer commonly presents as painless frank haematuria throughout the whole stream.

2) i.

This patient is describing (obstructive) voiding symptoms. In the eld-erly the most common cause would be BPH. At 29 years the most likely cause would be a urethral stricture especially with a past med-ical history of gonorrhoea which predisposes to stricture formation.

3) b.

This is a classical history of renal colic which can occur at any age, usu-ally middle age. It is more common in people who work or live in a hot environment because of dehydration. When the stone falls into the ureter the pain becomes colicky in nature radiating along the course of the ureter from loin to groin. Patients cannot get comfortable with their pain and are usually rolling around unable to keep still, unlike patients with peritonitis. Some have LUTS with nausea and vomitting.

4) f.

This lady has all the symptoms associated with a lower urinary tract infection. There is a peak in incidence around this age group due to ascending infection associated with sexual intercourse (honeymoon cystitis).

5) j.

These findings are consistent with a hydrocoele. As one can get above it, this rules out an inguinoscrotal hernia. Epidydimal cysts can be felt separate from the testicle, whereas in a hydrocoele the straw-coloured fluid surrounds the testicle completely making it impalpable and transilluminate brightly.

EMQ 2

a. Liver function tests
b. IVP
c. Echocardiogram
d. Laparoscopic radical nephrectomy
e. Embolisation of the tumour
f. Radical prostatectomy
g. Prostate specific antigen (PSA) blood test
h. Bladder biopsy
i. Transrectal ultrasound and prostate biopsy
j. Conservative management

Select the most appropriate treatment option or investigation for the patients described below:

1) A 55-year-old printer presents with recurrent UTI's and is found to have a red lesion in his bladder on flexible cystoscopy.

2) A 65-year-old Afro-Caribbean man presents worried that he might have prostate cancer. His younger brother has just been diagnosed with prostate cancer, which his father died of at the age of 70 years. On examination his prostate felt normal.

3) A fit 55-year-old woman presents having had two episodes of painless frank haematuria. The only abnormality detected during her haematuria screen was a $9 \times 8 \times 7$ cm solid mass in her right kidney seen on USS. The mass enhanced during a contrast CT scan.

4) A 72-year-old woman presents with painless frank haematuria.

5) A 24-year-old man presents with a six-hour history of colicky loin to groin pain. He is found to have a 4 mm ureteric calculus lodged in his left vesico-ureteric junction on non-contrast CT scan. There is no evidence of a urinary tract infection. His pain settles over the next few hours.

Answers

1) h.
A biopsy of the bladder lesion is the next appropriate step. This can be done at the time of the flexible cystoscopy or with a rigid cysto-scope under a general anaesthetic.

2) g.
This is a question about risk factors for prostate cancer of which he has two — being Afro-Caribbean and a positive family history. Although this man's prostate felt normal it does not rule out prostate cancer, as some cancers are not palpable on digital rectal examina-tion. PSA is much more sensitive at detecting prostate cancer and should be checked in view of his increased risk of prostate cancer.

3) d.
An enhancing solid renal mass seen on CT scan is diagnostic of malignant renal tumours. The treatment involves not just removing the kidney but also the surrounding perinephric fat within Gerota's fascia making it a radical as opposed to a simple nephrectomy. This is done laparoscopically where possible.

EMQ 3

a. Renal USS
b. Plain abdominal X-ray
c. Scrotal ultrasound scan
d. Renogram
e. CT scan
f. Antibiotics and analgesia
g. Emergency scrotal exploration
h. Nesbit procedure
i. Radical orchidectomy
j. Surgical ligation of the testicular vein(s)

Select the most appropriate option for the patients described below:

1) A 12-year-old boy presents having woken up from sleep with a very painful right testicle. The pain radiates into the groin and he is nauseous. On examination he has an exquisitely painful high riding testicle with a horizontal lie and an absent cremasteric reflex. Urinalysis was normal. He has had similar episodes in the past lasting for a few minutes.

2) A 24-year-old man presents with a hard painless testicular lump that has slowly increased in size over the past three months.

3) A 50-year-old man has his left testicle removed for a 2 × 2 × 3 cm testicular tumour. It is diagnosed as a germ cell cancer. Several months later he is feeling lethargic and generally run down.

4) A 70-year-old man presents with a two-day history of frequency, urgency, dysuria, and a painful swollen right testicle. One week earlier he had undergone

a TURP. On examination the overlying skin is red and hot, the testicle is generally enlarged and the epididymus is thickened. Urinalysis is positive for blood, leucocytes, nitrites and protein.

5) A 13-year-old boy presents with left sided scrotal swelling and a dull ache, which is worse at the end of the day. On palpation the left hemi scrotum has a fluctuant "bag of worms" surrounding a slightly small testicle. The swelling disappears when he lies flat. An USS confirms that it is a varicocoele with a normal left kidney.

Answers

1) g.
This is a classical history of testicular torsion the diagnosis of which is based on the history and examination. The management for any suspected torsion is emergency exploration, untwisting and bilateral fixation.

2) c.
The patient needs an urgent scrotal USS to see if it is a testicular tumour.

3) e.
He needs an urgent CT scan of his chest, abdomen and pelvis to rule out metastatic lymph node disease. Testicular cancer metastasises to the iliac, para- and pre-aortic lymph nodes as well as the lungs.

4) f.
This gentleman most likely has epididymo-orchitis, a recognised complication post-TURP. His urine should be sent for culture and sensitivity and he should be started on antibiotics and analgesics. A scrotal support is often helpful.

5) j.
Varicocoles are dilated veins around the testicle. They are occasionally associated with left renal tumours that are invading the left renal vein, obstructing the drainage of the testicular vein. Varicocoeles are only operated on if testicular growth is impaired, because of pain or large size or subfertility. The treatment is surgical ligation of the veins laparoscopically or as an open procedure or radiological embolisation.

EMQ 4

a. Trans-urethral resection of prostate (TURP)
b. LHRH analogue (Zoladex) or orchidectomy
c. Radiotherapy
d. Brachytherapy
e. Radical cystectomy
f. Extracorporeal shock wave lithotripsy (ESWL)
g. A 5-alpha reductase inhibitor
h. Ureteroscopy, fragmentation and basket removal of the calculus
i. Orchidopexy
j. Watchful waiting

Select the most appropriate treatment option for the patients described below:

1) A two-year-old boy is found to have a normal testicle palpable in the right inguinal canal and a normal left testicle in the scrotum.
2) A 48-year-old man has an 8 mm stone in the right renal pelvis. It is causing him moderate intermittent loin pain.
3) An 85-year-old man diagnosed with asymptomatic metastatic prostate cancer.
4) An airplane pilot presents with a one-week history of left loin to groin pain. He is diagnosed with a 7 mm stone at the VUJ. He is unable to work with this condition.
5) A 40-year-old man with significant LUTS is found to have BPH. He does not want surgery.

Answers

1) i.
An Orchidopexy involves freeing the testicle and cord from surrounding tissues and bringing the testicle down into the scrotum where it is placed in a subcutaneous "Dartos pouch". This needs to be done ideally before three years of age. It is usually done in one stage but sometimes needs to be done in two stages or transplanted down into the scrotum. The undescended testicle has an increased risk of developing cancer and needs to be examined regularly by the patient for the rest of his life.

2) f.
The treatment of choice would be non-invasive ESWL. The stone is fragmented by sound waves focused through the tissues onto the stone. Usually stones < 1.5 cm can be treated in this way.

3) b.

Prostate cancer growth is stimulated by testosterone. Treatment that reduces testosterone levels initially reduces the growth or shrinks most prostate cancers. This can be achieved by surgical castration (orchidectomy) or chemical castration using luteinising hormone releasing hormone (LHRH) analogues, or testosterone receptor blockers such as cyproterone acetate or bicalutamide (Casodex).

4) h.

In view of his job he needs early definitive treatment. The chance of the stone passing is about 60% at three weeks. As he is also in pain the best treatment option would be ureteroscopy, fragmentation and basket removal of the stone. Stones can be fragmented using a lithoclast or laser. ESWL, although an option, may take several treatment sessions to completely fragment the stone and sometimes days to pass the fragments.

5) g.

The 5-alpha reductase inhibitors shrink the size of the prostate gland, improving LUTS and reducing the likelihood of needing future surgery or developing acute urinary retention.

EMQ 5

a. Left colicky loin to groin pain
b. Left sided guarding on abdominal examination
c. Left renal mass
d. Pneumaturia
e. Leakage of urine on coughing
f. Storage symptoms (urgency, frequency, nocturia)
g. Left testicular pain
h. Urge urinary incontinence
i. Passage of a weak intermittent urinary stream
j. Continuous urinary incontinence

Suggest the most relevant symptom or sign from the above list for the following diagnosis:

1) A woman with a vesico-vaginal fistula.
2) A woman with a colo-vesical fistula.
3) A patient with superficial multifocal bladder cancer.

4) A patient with a left renal cell carcinoma.
5) A patient with stress urinary incontinence.

Answers

1) j.
A vesico-vaginal fistula is an abnormal connection between the vagina and bladder usually as a result of iatrogenic injury (surgery, radiotherapy). As a result there is a continuous leakage of urine into the vagina resulting in continuous urinary incontinence.

2) d.
A colo-vesical fistula usually occurs as a result of colonic cancer, diverticulitis, bladder cancer or radiotherapy. These patients often complain of passing debris (faeces) in the urine and suffer with recurrent UTI's. Often flatus from the bowel enters the urinary tract which is expelled as bubbles in the urine known as pneumaturia.

3) f.
Although bladder cancer is most commonly associated with haematuria, it can present with storage symptoms especially if the cancer covers a large surface area.

4) c.
Renal cell carcinomas were described as classically presenting with a triad of symptoms/signs which included flank pain, haematuria and an abdominal mass. Today this accounts for only 10% of cases. Most are detected as incidental finding on a scan for another condition.

5) e.
Leakage of urine on coughing or straining is known as stress urinary incontinence. It is usually as a result of childbirth and reflects a weakness of the pelvic floor muscles that support the bladder neck and urethra.

Chapter 12   Orthopaedics

Andrew Goldberg

Multiple Choice Questions

[Each single best answer (SBA) question comprises a stem and a number of answers. You are asked to decide which single item represents the best answer to the question.]

1. **The knee joint**

    a) Is a saddle joint
    b) Has two compartments
    c) Is stabilised by collateral ligaments
    d) Contains menisci made from hyaline cartilage
    e) Is supplied by the lateral cutaneous nerve of the thigh

[Best Answer = c]

Explanation

The knee joint is a condylar joint, where there is primarily movement in one plane (i.e. flexion, extension) with small amounts of movement in another plane (rotation). Some books also describe the knee as a hinge joint, which is not strictly true as hinge joints do not rotate. A saddle joint is only found at the carpometacarpal articulation of the thumb. The knee is divided into three compartments, the medial and lateral tibiofemoral joints and the patellofemoral articulation. The knee is stabilised on either side by the collateral ligaments and centrally by the cruciate ligaments. The articular surfaces are lined by hyaline (glass-like) cartilage, but the menisci are made of fibrocartilage, which as its name suggests is much more fibrous. The nerve supply to the knee follows Hilton's Law, which states that the nerve supply to a joint also tends to supply the muscles that move the joint or the skin that covers the muscles. For the knee that would be branches of the obturator, sciatic and femoral. It would not include the lateral cutaneous nerve as this is a superficial sensory nerve (L2,3).

2. The shoulder joint

a) Is a ball and socket joint
b) Is the most stable of all joints
c) Is supplied by the musculocutaneous nerve
d) Usually dislocates posteriorly
e) Dislocation is usually treated surgically

[Best Answer = a]

Explanation

The shoulder joint is a ball in socket joint, although it is a very shallow socket, and is reinforced by the glenoid labrum, a fibro-cartilaginous rim that increases the depth of the socket. Its nerve supply is from the axillary nerve. The shoulder is the most mobile of all the joints and as a result is the most unstable, especially infe-riorly where there is no cover by the rotator cuff. Almost all cases of dislocation of the shoulder are anterior dislocations (95%) and occur in abduction, external rotation (the position of throwing a baseball). Often the glenoid labrum is pulled off anteriorly, and this is called a Bankart lesion. If the humeral head impacts against the relatively hard anterior glenoid a defect can occur on the superior surface of the humeral head called a Hill Sachs lesion. This occurs in 35%–40% of anterior dislocations. A Hill Sachs lesion may destabilise the glenohumeral joint and predispose to further dislo-cation. There are a number of described manoeuvres to reduce an anterior dislocation, although the gentlest and kindest to the artic-ular surfaces involves just gentle traction, abduction and internal rotation. Surgery is usually reserved for those with a large Bankart lesion or a large Hill Sachs lesion that develop recurrent instability. There is a cohort of patients with a muscle patterning problem (essentially an unbalanced sequencing of muscle recruitment around the glenohumeral joint resulting in destabilisation) and sur-gery should be avoided in these patients.

3. Rheumatoid arthritis

a) Is an auto-immune disease
b) Usually affects the distal interphalangeal joints

c) Must be rheumatoid factor positive to confirm diagnosis
d) Can affect any fibrous joint
e) Is equal in incidence between men and women

[Best Answer = a]

Explanation

> Rheumatoid arthritis is an auto-immune disease that can affect any synovial joint and is more common in women. Whilst osteoarthritis tends to affect the distal IP joints (Heberden's nodes), RA tends to affect the proximal joints (MCP joints). Approximately 20% of patients with RA will be rheumatoid factor negative.

4. Greenstick fractures

a) Only occur in adolescents
b) Tend to buckle rather than break
c) Take twice as long to heal than complete fractures
d) Always need reduction
e) Must be investigated for non-accidental injury (NAI)

[Best Answer = b]

Explanation

> An immature bone is covered in a thick layer of periosteum and is much softer than adult bone. If you think of a young green twig (hence greenstick) compared to a dried out older brown twig. On bending the former buckles whilst the latter breaks in half. Children's fractures heal much faster than adult fractures and the younger the child, the quicker it takes to heal. A rough rule of thumb is to halve the time it takes for adults bones. NAI is a complex issue and relies on a number of indicators, in particular, the history given as well as the affect of the child. Other indicators are delay in presentation, unexplained injuries such as rib fractures or cigarette burn marks, or multiple injuries.

5. Pathological fractures

a) Occur in osteoarthritis
b) Always imply malignancy
c) Can occur in osteoporosis
d) Rarely occur without trauma
e) Always require internal fixation

[Best Answer = c]

Explanation

Pathological fractures are fractures occurring in a bone that has already been weakened by disease, and may occur at normal physiological stresses, without any trauma. There are many causes, including generalised bone diseases or metastatic deposits in the bone. One could think of pathological fractures as being of two types: one where a fracture occurs in a patient with generalised bone disease, such as a crushed vertebra or a fractured neck of femur in an osteoporotic lady; the other type occurs in patients with normal bone structure, but the fracture is in a localised area of abnormal bone, such as through a metastatic deposit. Although surgical fixation is often used, it is not mandatory and certain patients such as those with a non-weight bearing fracture might be better off with conservative treatment.

6. Fracture healing

a) Inflammation is an abnormal part of the healing process
b) Remodel according to the stresses the bone is subjected to
c) Torsional forces speed up healing
d) Is not affected by smoking
e) Is faster after internal fixation

[Best Answer = b]

Explanation

There are five stages to the healing of a fracture: bleeding, inflammation, proliferation, consolidation, and remodelling. Compression forces can increase the amount of callus, but twisting forces can prevent healing. There are two types of fracture healing: one is primary cortical healing and the other is periosteal bridging callus. Primary cortical healing is seen after rigid internal fixation and involves cutting cones travelling across the fracture akin to haversian remodelling. This is, if anything, a slower process than that seen in periosteal bridging callus, which is the method by which most fractures heal. Smoking, poor blood supply and infection reduce bone healing.

7. Fracture non-union

a) Is usually atrophic
b) Is differentiated from delayed union by X-ray appearances
c) Can be due to poor blood supply
d) Is less likely in smokers
e) Indicates the presence of infection

[Best Answer = c]

Explanation

Non-union has two characteristic X-ray appearances. Usually the bone ends look rounded (like elephant feet) and appear dense and sclerotic, and this is called hypertrophic non-union. In these cases there is plenty of new bone formation but for some reason the two ends do not unite (perhaps because of movement or interposed tissues). Less commonly, the bone can look osteopenic, and it is then called atrophic non-union, which is probably due to inadequate blood supply. Smoking is known to inhibit bone healing and the risk of non-union is therefore much higher in smokers. Whilst infection can cause a non-union, of course a non-union does not imply infection.

There is no absolute exact distinction in terms of the time when you should describe a fracture as non union as opposed to delayed union as opposed to; however, if the bone has failed to unite after several months, it is unlikely to heal without intervention and is usually described as non-union.

8. Sudek's atrophy (complex regional pain syndrome type I)

a) Can present with discolouration
b) Bone scans are required for diagnosis
c) The limb must be immobilised
d) A sympathectomy should usually be carried out
e) Has a worse prognosis in children

[Best Answer = a]

Explanation

Sudek's atrophy can lead to a blue or pale, cold limb as a result of vasoconstriction or redness and warmth as a result of capillary vasodilation. Livedo reticularis (a purplish mottling) of the extremity has also been described. Diagnosis is mainly based on clinical findings although a three-phase bone scan can be a useful adjunct, with abnormalities noted on the delayed image (after 30 minutes) which shows increased periarticular activity. However the bone scan is said to only be sensitive within the first three to six months, after which it is much less useful. Treatment is usually conservative, with counselling, pain management and physical therapy although sympathectomy is sometimes helpful. Immobility tends to make the condition worse and prognosis is better in children compared to adults.

9. Salter-Harris injuries

a) Involve the diaphysis
b) In adults have a better prognosis
c) Always involve the joint surface
d) Can lead to growth disturbance
e) Always require open reduction and internal fixation

[Best Answer = d]

Explanation

Injuries at the physeal end of long bones of children can be categorised according to the Salter-Harris Classification. This classification is not relevant to mature bones without a growth plate (physis). Salter-Harris III and IV injuries involve the joint surface. Any injury involving the physis can potentially lead to growth disturbance. The worst fractures are the ones where a growth plate injury, such as a crush, is missed at the time of the injury (e.g. Salter-Harris V) and are not picked up until growth is distorted. Whilst intra-articular epiphyseal injuries are usually treated by open reduction and internal fixation (ORIF), most other childhood fractures in children can be treated by manipulation under anaesthetic and then immobilisation in plaster.

10. Anterior cruciate ligament rupture

a) Usually results in a haemarthrosis
b) Necessitates surgery
c) Giving way is an indication for conservative treatment
d) Repair restores completely normal knee function
e) Repair has been shown to significantly reduce the risk of arthritis

[Best Answer = a]

Explanation

A torn anterior cruciate ligament (ACL) invariably leads to a haemarthrosis, and a knee injury with a haemarthrosis should be considered an ACL rupture until proven otherwise. The treatment after rupture of the ACL may be operative or conservative. Approximately a third of patients can develop sufficient stability without the need for surgery mainly through muscular training and education. If, despite physical therapy, a patient continues to suffer from "giving way" then an ACL repair operation should be recommended to attempt to restore stability, although the proprioceptive function of the ACL is often lost or reduced and so surgery cannot restore completely normal knee function.

In the US over 50,000 ACL reconstructions take place each year, nonetheless, we do not really know if surgery prevents longer term arthititis. It is logical to assume that an unstable knee has a higher chance of developing osteoarthritis earlier than the same knee with an intact ACL. The confounding factors include other injuries, such as meniscal tears and damage to the articular surfaces at the time of injury. Also further injuries sustained subsequently (especially if the individual returns to sports) will further confound the long term results of any ACL repair. The definitive answer to the question, "will an ACL repair prevent me from getting osteoarthritis?" may never be found.

11. Total hip replacement

a) Has a 60% success rate
b) Usually leaves the operated leg short
c) Deep infection occurs in 5%
d) DVT is prevented by heparin
e) Polyethylene wear debris is a cause of aseptic loosening

[Best Answer = e]

Explanation

Total hip replacement (THR) is a very successful procedure for arthritis of the hip with a good result in about 95% of cases. Most surgeons aim to restore leg length so there is no discrepancy with the opposite side, although studies have shown that if there is a leg length discrepancy, it tends to leave the operated leg longer rather than shorter. Anything greater than 1 cm is likely to make the patient symptomatic. The incidence of deep wound infection has been reported to be about 1% although the incidence of superficial wound infection is much higher. Studies have shown that up to 50% of THR's suffer a DVT and the risk is approximately halved with heparin prophylaxis, although no prophylaxis can prevent DVT completely. Polyethylene wear debris, which is formed by the rubbing of the head on the polyethylene liner, has been implicated in aseptic loosening. The particles which are of a similar size to bacteria are phagocytosed by macrophages and this can lead to an inflammatory reaction and eventually aseptic loosening of the prosthesis.

12. Total knee replacements

a) Results are less satisfactory than hip replacements
b) Have a high incidence of DVT
c) Are lighter than the resected bone
d) Foot drop is a common complication
e) Playing golf after a TKR is contra-indicated

[Best Answer = b]

Explanation

The success rate of this operation is as good as THR. In the UK a register of hip and knee replacements was introduced in 2002 but data from overseas suggests a good knee replacement in a compliant patient should last 15–20 years.

The materials used for the prostheses include titanium alloys, cobalt-chrome or stainless steel, and these tend to be heavier than the resected bone. As for THR, complications include DVT, which occurs in about 50%–75% of TKR's (the incidence is halved if heparin prophylaxis is used).

The common peroneal nerve travels around the fibular neck and can be injured during retraction. This can lead to foot drop and although a rare complication, should be mentioned as part of the consenting process. Many patients with a TKR have returned to playing golf without any problems.

13. The radial nerve

a) Comes off the medial cord of the brachial plexus
b) Is predominantly a sensory nerve
c) Injury leads to loss of extension of the metarcarpophalangeal joints
d) Injury in the radial groove leads to loss of elbow extension
e) The anterior interosseous nerve supplies all finger extensors

[Best Answer = c]

Explanation

The radial nerve (C6,7,8) comes of the posterior cord of the brachial plexus. The radial nerve is predominantly a motor nerve. It is the nerve which extends the fingers, the wrist and the elbow. Injury at the level of the radial groove, will lead to a wrist drop and loss of extension at the MCPJ's but not loss of extension of the elbow, because the triceps receives its innervation more proximally. **Note:** When testing finger extension in a patient with a backslab on, it is important to look for extension of the MCPJ's rather than just extension of the PIPJ's, which can be accomplished by the lumbricals, which are not supplied by the radial nerve. The posterior interosseous nerve is a branch of the radial nerve and supplies all finger extensors. Note that the anterior interosseous is a branch of the median nerve and not related to the radial nerve.

14. Carpal tunnel syndrome

a) Is caused by compression of the ulnar nerve
b) Is associated with rheumatoid arthritis
c) Patients have pain in the little and ring fingers
d) Can lead to weakness of the hypothenar muscles
e) Should be definitively treated with a steroid injection

[Best Answer = b]

Explanation

Carpal tunnel syndrome is caused by compression of the median nerve under the thick flexor retinaculum. It is associated with pregnancy, rheumatoid arthritis, hypothyroidism, acromegaly and trauma, although most often it is idiopathic in menopausal women. The classic symptoms are pain and paraesthesia in the distribution of the median nerve, namely, the volar aspect of the thumb, index and middle fingers. A small patch of skin over the thenar eminence is spared, because this is supplied by the superficial branch of the median nerve, which does not go under the flexor retinaculum. Treatment is by surgical decompression — division of the flexor retinaculum. Certain mild cases can be treated conservatively by using splints across the wrist and occasionally by a local anaesthetic and steroid injection.

15. The ulnar nerve

a) Is a branch of the lateral cord of the brachial plexus
b) Supplies the intrinsic muscles of the hand
c) Palsy causes wrist drop
d) The autonomous zone is the tip of the index finger
e) A positive Froment's sign indicates a functioning nerve

[Best Answer = b]

Explanation

The ulnar nerve (C8, T1) is a branch of the medial cord of the brachial plexus. Its sensory fibres supply the outer one and a half fingers (little and ring) and its autonomous zone is the tip of the little finger. The motor fibres supply all of the interossei, half of the flexor digitorum profundus (FDP) and the lumbricals to the ring and little fingers. Damage to the ulnar nerve usually occurs at the elbow or the wrist. The usual picture is a "claw-like hand". A lesion at the wrist causes unopposed action of the extensors and the FDP, especially of the little and ring fingers, causing them to claw (the FDP is supplied just below the elbow and so a cut at the level of the wrist will not paralyse this). Lesions at the elbow often have less clawing (known as the ulnar paradox), since the ulnar half of FDP is now paralysed and the fingers are therefore straighter. By asking the patient to grip a piece of paper between the thumb and the proximal phalanx of the index finger of a closed fist, one can test adductor pollicis. In an ulnar nerve lesion the patient is unable to use adductor pollicis, and to cheat they flex the DIPJ using the flexor pollicis (supplied by the median nerve). If they flex the DIPJ, then this is called a positive Froment's sign.

Case Studies

Case 1

A 76-year-old type II diabetic woman presents with a two-year history of progressive groin pain. She walks with a limp and has to stop after about 200 yards. She finds it difficult to put on her shoes and get in and out of a bath. She is on warfarin for a previous deep vein thrombosis.

a) What is the most likely diagnosis and what are the characteristics of this disease?

b) What investigations should be carried out?

c) What radiographic changes would you expect to see?

d) What is the management of her condition?

e) What are the most common complications of her treatment?

f) What risk factors does she have for these complications and what preventative measures could be taken to lower their risk?

Answers

a) The most likely diagnosis is that of osteoarthritis (OA) of her hip, which is a degenerative joint disorder in which there is progressive loss of articular cartilage in synovial joints. OA can be *primary*, where there is no obvious underlying cause, or *secondary*, when it follows a pre-existing abnormality of the joint (e.g. rheumatoid disease). Pain and capsular fibrosis usually account for the joint stiffness in osteoarthritis. Swellings in the fingers (Heberden's nodes at the distal interphalangeal joints and Bouchard's nodes at the PIPJ's) points to primary osteoarthritis. Osteoarthritis of the hip commonly presents with groin pain.

b) The most useful investigation is a plain AP radiograph of the pelvis and lateral of the affected hip. If surgery was to be contemplated then aside from routine blood tests one would need to look at diabetic compliance and in her case obtain a clotting screen to check her INR (she is on warfarin).

c) The common radiographic changes you would look for are narrowing of the joint space (as the cartilage is worn away); osteophytes (bits of bone overgrowth, usually near the edge of the joint); subchondral sclerosis; subchondral bone cysts; and eventually, structural damage.

d) In the early stages of the disease, treatment is conservative, using analgesics, weight loss, advice on altering load-bearing activities and physiotherapy to help increase joint mobility and strengthen the muscles. If conservative measures fail then the next step is a total joint replacement. Whilst the books also talk of osteotomies and arthorodesis, they tend to be tried in the young and so are not applicable in this lady.

e) The specific complications of a hip replacement include, leg length discrepancy, infection, dislocation, nerve injury (leading to foot drop) and loosening. General complications include bleeding, thromboembolism, chest infection, UTI, MI and death.

f) She has had a DVT in the past and is on warfarin. As a result she is at risk of bleeding intra-operatively. Assuming the warfarin will be stopped in advance of the surgery then she is at risk of a further DVT or PE. Invariably this is managed by the use of heparin, foot pumps and/or thromboembolic stockings and early mobilisation. In some cases a vena caval filter can be used pre-operatively. The other risk is her diabetes, which increases her risk of infection and myocardial infarction. The best prevention is optimisation of her diabetes and weight loss.

Case 2

A 13-year-old boy presents with a limp and right hip pain. He is tall and thin and has had a limp intermittently for the past six months.

a) What is the likely diagnosis?
b) What is the differential diagnosis?
c) What investigations should be performed?
d) What are the risk factors for this condition?
e) What would your initial management be?
f) What are the complications of this condition?

Answers

a) At his age the concern is a slipped capital femoral epiphysis (SCFE).

b) Any painful hip should set your mind thinking of a series of age related differentials. In the newborn, one should consider developmental dysplasia (DDH); between the ages of four to ten years, think of Perthes; and between the ages of ten years to maturity think of SCFE. Obviously the differential that must always be on your mind is infection, whether it is with a purulent organism or a viral infection (transient synovitis).

c) The investigations include a bedside temperature measurement, blood tests (which should include a white cell count, a CRP and an ESR), and radiographs. You should request an AP of the pelvis and a frog lateral X-ray to see both hips and be able to compare them. In the case of SCFE, you are looking for displacement of the femoral epiphysis from its normal position on the neck of the femur. It is a slight misnomer to call this slipped epiphysis, as the epiphysis stays in the acetabulum and if anything the neck of the femur slips anteriorly. Nonetheless, the end result is that the epiphysis is usually posteriorly located in relation to the neck.

d) SCFE tends to affect two contrasting groups, one being the fat and sexually underdeveloped group and the other being the tall and thin group — boys more than girls. Mechanical factors might play a part, since fat children have a higher incidence as may endocrine factors. One theory is that SCFE might be due to a hormonal imbalance at the time of a growth spurt.

e) Your initial management is to ensure that you are not missing infection. The best indicators are a raised temperature and raised inflammatory markers. If the temperature and the blood markers are normal, then your index of suspicion for infection can be lowered. Whilst the classification used to be broken down into acute or chronic, the current convention is to refer to SCFE as stable or unstable. If the patient is limping or in pain when walking, then by definition they have an unstable SCFE and require operative treatment. The patient should be advised to use crutches to prevent weight bearing, and at the next available opportunity they should have surgery to prevent any further slippage. Invariably, two or three cannulated screws are placed up the neck and into the epiphysis (*in situ* pinning) to prevent any further displacement. There is controversy about whether the displaced epiphysis should be reduced before it is pinned.

f) Most experts would agree that attempted reduction leads to a higher chance of chondrolysis, where the articular cartilage can break down at a later date. Although this can occur without surgery the risk is higher if the guide wire or pin penetrate the articular cartilage. Longer term these patients probably have a higher incidence of osteoarthritis, obviously the earlier the problem is picked up and treated the lower the risk.

Case 3

A one-week-old baby is sent with her parents to the orthopaedic clinic by the paediatrician who noticed uneven groin creases and asymmetrical abduction on clinical examination.

a) What is the most likely diagnosis?
b) What clinical tests would you carry out to confirm your diagnosis?
c) What other investigations would you carry out?
d) What is your initial management?
e) What are the risk factors for this condition?

Answers

a) The most likely diagnosis is that of congenital dislocation of the hip although nowadays the word congenital is rarely used in favour of the term DDH or developmental dysplasia of the hip.

b) Two clinical tests are used to diagnose the condition. **Ortolani's test** detects a dislocated hip (hint: "O" for out). The hips and knees are flexed to 90° and the thighs are grasped in each hand, the thumb over the inner thigh and the index finger resting over the greater trochanters. The hips are abducted gently and a resistance to abduction will be noted if the hip is dislocated, otherwise they abduct easily to 90°. When gentle pressure is applied to the greater trochanters by the index finger, a dislocated hip will relocate back into the joint and a click can be felt (positive Ortolani test). **Barlow's test** is a slight modification of this test. It is performed as above except during the abduction phase; gentle but firm pressure is applied in the line of the femur so that a lax hip dislocates posteriorly. The hip can then be reduced by performing the movement in Ortolani's test. Therefore, one could think of it as Ortolani's test detects a dislocated hip and Barlow's test detects a dislocatable hip.

c) If either of the above tests are positive, or your clinical index of suspicion is high then the baby should have an ultrasound scan. This will show the shape of the cartilaginous socket and the position of the head of the femur. X-rays are not helpful as the femoral head is not yet calcified.

d) Management aims to reduce the hip and hold the head of the femur in this position until the acetabular rim is sufficiently developed. Reduction can be obtained by closed or open methods. The younger the patient the more likely that closed methods will be possible. In the newborn this can be achieved initially with double nappies to abduct the hips, followed by a re-assessment after two to three weeks with another ultrasound examination. If the hip remains unstable it is possible to apply a special harness to hold the legs abducted. The most popular is called the Pavlik harness, which holds the legs in a position for a few months. It is imperative to check that the femoral head is in the right place using regular ultrasound. If after another month the hip will not remain reduced using a harness or spica, then it will be necessary to perform an examination under anaesthesia, probably with an arthrogram (dye injected into the joint) to look for concentricity of the hip and any anatomical abnormalities. If surgery is required you should just know some of the options, which include a tenotomy and/or derotation varus osteotomy. The patient should be followed up regularly with ultrasound examinations and once older than six months with radiographs.

e) The incidence of DDH is about two per 1000 live births although somewhere between five to 20 per 1000 hips are lax at birth. Females are affected more than males and one-third are bilateral. The exact aetiology is unknown but there is a familial tendency and there is a high incidence of both joint laxity and a shallow acetabulum in first order relatives of DDH patients. The position of the foetus in the uterus may play a part as there is a higher incidence in breech presentation, first born and those with oligohydramnios, all of which result in decreased intrauterine space. It is also interesting to note that the incidence is much higher in North

American Indians, who wrap their babies tight to the mother's body with the hips extended and the legs together, compared to the racially identical Eskimos, who carry their babies on the back with the hips widely abducted and flexed.

Case 4

A 78-year-old woman presents to A&E, following a fall, with pain in her hip and is unable to walk. She has a shortened externally rotated leg.

a) What is the most likely diagnosis?
b) What are the risk factors for this condition?
c) What is your management of this patient?
d) Why is her leg shortened and externally rotated?
e) What are the best predictors for prognosis in this condition?

Answers

a) The most likely diagnosis is a fracture of the neck of the femur, which is a loose term, probably better described as a fracture of the proximal femur.

b) Risk factors relate to trauma and the inherent strength of the underlying bones. Therefore osteoporosis which weakens bone quality, is the biggest risk factor, and hence the older the patient the higher the risk. Repeated falls, is obviously another risk factor.

c) The management of a patient with a hip fracture involves:

- Obtain a good history and social status for the patient.
- Insert a cannulae and send off bloods for U&E's, FBC and a group and save.
- Get an ECG and a chest X-ray and an X-ray of the pelvis and affected limb.
- If necessary, correct any medical problems (they are usually dehydrated and require fluid resuscitation), optimising them for theatre.
- Ensure the surgeon obtains informed consent and marks the limb.
- Prescribe anti-thromboembolism treatment (e.g. TED stockings, low molecular weight heparin or foot pumps).

- If the patient is in severe discomfort skin traction can be applied to reduce the pain.

The decision on which type of surgery is suitable, depends on whether the fracture is intracapsular or extracapsular and displaced or undisplaced. If the fracture is extracapsular, they will usally be treated by a dynamic hip screw (DHS) or a proximal femoral nail (PFN). If the fracture is intracapsular, then the treatment option is either to reduce the head and fix it with screws or to replace it. Remember the blood supply to the head of the femur travels up the neck and so displaced intra-articular fractures are at high risk of avascular necrosis and in these cases in the elderly, a hemiarthroplasty or hip replacement is currently the treatment of choice.

d) The leg is externally rotated and shortened because of the powerful iliopsoas muscle which is attached to the lesser trochanter of the femur. If the fracture is proximal to this attachment, then the pull of this muscle causes the affected limb to lie shortened and externally rotated.

e) These fractures have a high mortality (up to 40% at one year) no matter what treatment is performed in the initial period. The exact reason for this high mortality is unclear (even if you take into account the age and co-existing medical problems). The strongest predictors of outcome include mental state, pre-morbidity and mobility. Hence a patient who was alert and independent, who mobilised without any aids, is likely to have a good prognosis. On the other hand a patient with Alzheimer's, who was living in a nursing home and was wheelchair-bound will have a very poor prognosis.

Case 5

A 32-year-old male is brought into casualty following a road traffic accident. He was a pedestrian whose right leg was run over by a car at slow speed. He is alert and orientated. His vital signs are all normal but his left shin has a large wound and the bone is sticking through the wound.

a) What diagnosis are you expecting regarding his left leg?
b) What is your initial management in A&E?
c) What will be your management in theatre?

d) What are the principles of the definitive treatment?

e) What early complications are you most worried about?

Answers

a) This is an open fracture of his left tibia in a major trauma patient. Because a car went over his leg, a crush injury is suspected as well.

b) Any major trauma must be treated according to the Advanced Trauma Life Support (ATLS®) guidelines. It is important to deal with life-threatening injuries first. The airway (and cervical spine control), breathing, and circulation (ABC) take priority over the fracture. This all takes place as part of the primary survey, where trauma X-rays are also taken (C-spine, a chest and a pelvic X-ray). The fracture is usually assessed in the secondary (or top-to-toe) survey. Analgesia should be given and gross contaminants should be removed from the wound. If the patient has not received tetanus immunisation (i.e. tetanus toxoid) or their immunity is in question, then a booster should be given. Note that a booster does not provide immediate protection; hence we always start patients with open fractures on broad spectrum antibiotics as soon as possible (not waiting till they have gone to theatre), which cover for Staphylococcus, anaerobes and Clostridia. If the immunity of the patient is uncertain and the wound is very dirty then immunoglobulins can also be given, which give immediate protection. A photograph should be taken so that the wound does not need to be inspected repeatedly, and then the wound should be covered with an antiseptic-soaked dressing. If the limb is deformed then the leg can be straightened under sedation and splinted until the patient gets to theatre. It is of vital importance to check the neurovascular status both before and after any manipulation and the results documented in the notes. As this is an open fracture it is a surgical emergency and should be booked for theatre within six hours to prevent muscle necrosis.

c) In theatre, the wound is thoroughly washed out and any contaminated or dead tissue is debrided. The fracture is assessed and stabilised (usually by internal or external fixation). If the wound is large and primary closure is unlikely to be achieved, then a plastic surgeon should ideally be present in theatre, as it may be possible to perform a skin graft or flap procedure (alternatively the wound can be left open and re-inspected at about 48 hours for delayed primary closure or a skin grafting procedure).

d) The principles of the treatment of any fracture are the 4 R's — Resuscitation, Reduction, Restriction (immobilisation), and Rehabilitation. In particular in this case it is of vital importance to ensure the wound heals (i.e. good skin coverage), that infection is avoided, that the fracture heals in a good position and that the patient is rehabilitated to as good as function as possible.

e) The complications that are of most concern are neurovascular injury, compartment syndrome and infection. Given that this was a crush injury, compartment syndrome is of a particular worry. The best and earliest sign of compartment syndrome is pain on passive stretching of the muscles of the affected compartment (for the lower leg there are four compartments — please learn these). Although compartment pressures can be useful, especially in an unconscious patient, diagnosis is in the main made on clinical findings and in particular pain that is out of proportion to clinical findings. If you look for the six P's of acute ischaemia, you might be misled, because, the pulses usually do not disappear until late. In addition, the limb is often warm and red rather than cold and clammy. The limb is usually tense and the veins are often engorged. Surgical decompression (where the tight fascia of each of the compartments is divided to relieve the pressure on the muscles) must be within six hours otherwise irreversible damage will result.

Extended Matching Questions

EMQ 1

a. Closed or open reduction and internal fixation
b. Hemiarthroplasty
c. Total hip replacement
d. Hip resurfacing
e. Arthrodesis
f. Traction
g. Physical therapy
h. Plaster of Paris
i. External fixation
j. Removable splint
k. Manipulation under anaesthetic

Select the most appropriate definitive treatment option for the patients described below:

1) A 75-year-old man who is referred to the clinic by his GP with a year's history of groin pain. Examination reveals an irritable hip with a reduced range of movement and his radiograph shows advanced joint space narrowing, osteophytes and subchondral sclerosis.
2) An 89-year-old lady who is brought into the A&E from a nursing home following a fall. Her leg is shortened and externally rotated and the radiograph demonstrates an inter-trochanteric fracture.
3) A 37-year-old man presents to the clinic with a two-day history of pain in his right buttock radiating down his right thigh, especially worse on coughing or sneezing or bending forwards.
4) A baby girl aged 18 months has fallen off a swing and is brought to the A&E with pain and deformity in her thigh.
5) A 90-year-old right-handed lady presents to the A&E following a fall onto an outstretched hand. She has a dinner fork deformity.

Answers

1) c.
The most likely diagnosis is osteoarthritis of the hip. Assuming the GP has tried conservative measures such as analgesics, weight loss, and physical therapy and surgical intervention is needed, a total hip

replacement would be the definitive treatment of choice as it has such good results. Hip resurfacing is increasing in popularity with younger patients, with good short term results but is not yet the accepted mainstay of treatment until long term data/results become available.

2) a.

She may have been lying on the floor for some time and is likely to be dehydrated. Initial management involves fluid resuscitation and analgesia. If there is a delay until theatre, the application of skin traction might help distract the fracture ends and reduce the pain but is not a definitive treatment (as being bed bound for six weeks has many complications). Surgical treatment is closed reduction and internal fixation. A dynamic hip screw and plate (DHS) is the current treatment of choice. A hemiarthroplasty is not required as the blood supply to the head is usually intact.

3) g.

The most likely diagnosis is that of mechanical back pain. The usual cause of lower back pain is muscular spasm although the history of worsening on bending forwards is suggestive of possible disc pathology. A bulging disc is caused by micro-tears of the annulus fibrosis leading to weakness and a bulge of the contents of the disc. If the annulus tears properly, then the disc can prolapse into the spinal canal. The pressure on the nerve roots (and associated chemical inflammation) causes "sciatica" which is a shooting pain down the distribution of the sciatic nerve. Treatment involves analgesia and rest initially. Once the acute pain has settled, it is important that the patient mobilises as much as possible as rest can simply make the muscle spasm worse. Hence advice and physiotherapy are indicated. In particular exercises to strengthen the "core stabilising" muscles are said to be important. Surgery should be avoided unless there is progressive neurology, which would warrant an MRI scan in the first instance.

4) f.

The most likely diagnosis is that of a displaced fractured femur. Undisplaced fractures can be treated in a plaster spica on presentation although displaced fractures in a child weighing less than 15 kg are usually treated with Gallows traction. This is fixed traction against the weight of the child's body. Both the fractured and the opposite femur are placed in skin traction and the child is suspended by these from a special frame. Both the legs are held vertically in the air, with the child's torso remaining on the bed. The buttocks should be just off the bed. Vascular compromise is the biggest danger and the circulation should be checked frequently. Adequate analgesia is important. It is not suitable for children weighing greater than 15 kg as too much force will be applied to the skin, which can be damaging. The Gallows traction remains on for two to three weeks and when the child starts wriggling about in the bed, you know the fracture is healing and you might consider replacing it with a plaster spica.

5) k.
The most likely diagnosis is a Colles' fracture or fracture of the distal radius. A dinner fork deformity results from shortening and dorsal angulation of the distal fragment. The usual treatment in this case would be closed reduction (manipulation under anaesthesia) followed by immobilisation in a plaster. The plaster would remain on for about five to six weeks. If the fracture was grossly unstable or involved the joint surface then some form of fixation such as K-wires, an external fixator or open reduction and internal fixation would be alternative options.

EMQ 2

a. Osteoarthritis
b. Osteomalacia
c. Osteoporosis
d. Metastases
e. Infection
f. Open fracture
g. Primary bone tumour
h. Rheumatoid arthritis
i. Traction apophysitis
j. Paget's disease

Select the most appropriate diagnosis for the patients described below:

1) A 73-year-old man presents with a three-year history of pain in his right hip and thigh. He also complained that his hat no longer fits.
2) A 36-year-old Somalian man presents with a two-month history of lower back pain. He has recent weight loss and night sweats.

3) A 72-year-old lady presents with lower back pain after a fall. In her past medical history she was noted to have had a fractured wrist and a fractured neck of femur.

4) A ten-year-old girl presents with a two-month history of thigh pain and a swelling that is gradually increasing in size. Her pain keeps her up at night.

5) A 60-year-old man presents with a stiff, painful and swollen knee. Fifteen years ago he had a fracture of his tibial plateau that was treated with open reduction and internal fixation.

Answers

1) j.
The most likely diagnosis is Paget's disease, also known as osteitis deformans. In Paget's there is a malfunction in the normal process of bone remodelling with an increase in bone resorption (osteoclasts) and a compensatory increase in bone formation (osteoblasts). The resultant bone is disorganised, abnormal and mechanically weak. Paget's disease can affect any bone, but the common sites are the skull, the pelvis and femurs. Because Paget's bones have an increased blood supply, the patient can also suffer high output cardiac failure. Many patients are asymptomatic. If symptoms are present, they tend to be pain and later deformity. Other presentations include, pathological fracture, spinal stenosis, deafness or an increased skull size, where the patient may note that their hat no longer fits. Alkaline phosphatase is usually raised and can be a marker for treatment, which involves drugs to reduce osteoclastic activity (bisphosphonates). Rarely Paget's patients can develop an osteosarcoma.

2) e.
The most likely diagnosis is that of mechanical back pain, however, the symptoms of weight loss and night sweats raises the concern for an infective process, of which TB would be high on the list, especially in view of his country of origin.

3) c.
The most likely diagnosis here is an osteoporotic vertebral crush fracture, in which the body of the vertebrae collapses due to compression and flexion. This typically happens in post-menopausal osteoporotics where the bone is weak and sometimes occurs under normal physiological loads.

4) g.

Any child with a history of greater than six weeks pain, especially if the pain occurs at night is worrying. Bone tumours can be benign or malignant and can arise from any of the tissues that make up the bone, including cartilage, bone, periosteum, fibrous tissue or marrow. In a ten-year-old, an osteosarcoma and Ewing's tumour must be on the differential.

5) a.

The most likely diagnosis is osteoarthritis. A tibial plateau fracture is an intra-articular fracture and increases the risk of developing subsequent osteoarthritis. The painful swollen knee could be an acute monoarthritis although infection cannot be ruled out on the history alone. Blood tests and culture of the joint fluid will give a definitive diagnosis.

EMQ 3

a. Sudek's atrophy (complex regional pain syndrome type I)
b. Avascular necrosis
c. Frozen shoulder
d. Carpal tunnel syndrome
e. Ruptured extensor pollicis longus
f. Malunion
g. Non-union
h. Foot drop
i. Wrist drop
j. Myositis ossificans
k. Growth disturbance

Select the most likely complication for the patients described below:

1) A 40-year-old lady comes out of plaster after eight weeks, following treatment of an ankle fracture. Her foot is swollen, red, sweaty and painful.
2) A 64-year-old patient who has been treated in plaster for six weeks for a Colles fracture and has a dinner fork deformity.
3) A patient who suffered a knee dislocation playing football and post-reduction finds they drag their foot on the floor when walking.
4) A 56-year-old patient who had an intracapsular fractured neck of femur treated by closed reduction and cannulated screws.
5) A patient who was immobilised with a sling for four weeks for a fracture of his radial neck and now has stiffness of the elbow.

Answers

1) a.

This condition also used to be called post-traumatic osteodystrophy. It is usually not noticed until the plaster has been removed, several weeks after the injury. The cause is thought to be due to autonomic changes with an unusual sympathetic response. If there is no associated nerve damage then the condition is called **CRPS type 1**. If there is associated nerve damage then it is **CRPS type 2.** It often looks and feels like infection, which is obviously a differential diagnosis. Although the condition is usually self-limiting, some patients find it disabling and need the care of the anaesthetic pain specialists. Guanethidine nerve blocks and sympathectomy seem to help in some cases.

2) f.

Colles described an extra-articular fracture of the distal radius (within an inch and a half of the joint). These fractures can occur at any age after a fall onto an outstretched hand, however, are most common in the elderly with osteoporosis. There is usually dorsal angulation and radial deviation of the distal fragment and because the fragments are impacted there is also shortening. The above displacement is usually called a "dinner fork" deformity as that is what it looks like. Reduction aims to restore length and correct the dorsal angulation, although sometimes in plaster the deformity recurs which is likely to have occurred in this patient (either that or it was never reduced in the first place). There are a number of other uncommon but well described complications following a Colles fracture including Sudek's atrophy; adhesive capsulitis of the (frozen) shoulder — due to immobility; carpal tunnel syndrome and rupture of the tendon of extensor pollicis longus (note that the tendon hooks around Lister's tubercle which is where it is susceptible to increased friction against a sharp bony fragment and the patient usually presents with an inability to extend their thumb several weeks after the injury).

3) h.

The common peroneal nerve travels around the neck of the fibula and studies suggest that it is injured in approximately 20% of patients who suffer a traumatic knee dislocation. Injury to the nerve leads to weakness of ankle and toe dorsiflexors and the gait is sometimes referred to as steppage gait, because the hip and knee flexors have to overwork to prevent the toes from catching on the ground during the swing phase.

4) b.

The femoral head receives its major blood supply from vessels that travel under the capsule and up the neck. In displaced intracapsular fractures this blood supply can be damaged leading to the risk of subsequent avascular necrosis which usually presents as groin pain and can take up to 18 months to be visible on X-rays. The more displaced the fracture, the higher the risk of avascular necrosis and for Garden IV fractures (complete displacement) the risk can be as high as 80% or higher. The incidence of non-union ranges from 10%–30% in different studies.

5) j.

Elbow injuries are notorious for developing stiffness, even after relatively innocuous injuries. The incidence varies in the literature from 5% to 38% post-fracture dislocation. Stiffness can either be caused by extrinsic pathology such as capsular scarring or myositis ossificans (calcification of the soft tissues) or intrinsic pathology where the articular surfaces are injured and there is a bony block to movement. In most cases, the cause is a mixture of intrinsic and extrinsic pathology.

EMQ 4

a. Ganglion
b. Dupytrens disease
c. Trigger finger
d. Carpal tunnel syndrome
e. Osgood schlatter's disease
f. Bone cyst
g. Lipoma
h. Fibroma
i. Inclusion dermoid
j. Sebaceous cyst

Select the most likely diagnosis for the patients described below:

1) A 56-year-old man presents to a clinic with a flexion deformity of his ring and little finger.

2) A 32-year-old patient presents with a lump on the dorsum that transilluminates to light.

3) A 12-year-old boy with a painful lump in the front of his knee, just below the kneecap, worse after exercise.

4) A 14-year-old boy who presents to casualty following a knee sprain and an asymptomatic lytic lesion is noted in the femur on X-ray.

5) A 56-year-old lady complains that her middle finger gets caught flexed and is painful.

Answers

1) b.
Dupuytren's is a disorder where there is fibrosis and thickening of the palmar fascia (not the tendons!) The aetiology is not known, although it can be inherited as an autosomal dominant gene. The associations include alcohol, drugs (such as phenytoin), cirhossis and diabetes. Surgery is considered for progressive lesions where the hand can no longer be placed flat on a table, which in mild cases may take years. It usually involves a fasciectomy, where the palmar fascia is divided and excised. Because the digital nerve sits within the fascia it is clearly at risk during surgery.

2) a.
The origins of a ganglion are debated but is probably a cystic mucoid degeneration of the joint capsule or tendon sheath. The most common location is around the wrist. If found in the palm, in the region of the metarcapophalangeal joints, they are called a pearl ganglion. A ganglion can disappear spontaneously, although a bash with a Bible was the traditional treatment. It is smooth and fluctuant and those at the wrist are usually fixed to deeper structures but not to skin. It can be aspirated (thick, gel-like material) and injected with hydrocortisone, although it commonly recurs, in which case it can be surgically excised.

3) e.
Osgood-Schlatter's disease is a traction apophysitis of the insertion of the patellar tendon on the tibial tuberosity that occurs in adolescents during growth spurt (boys more than girls). The condition was described by two separate surgeons in the same year (1903). Most cases are treated conservatively with rest, painkillers and physiotherapy and it

is typically a self-limited condition that waxes and wanes, but invariably resolves although this process can take months to years to resolve entirely. In recalcitrant cases surgical debridement and removal of bony ossicles behind the tendon can have a good result.

4) f.

Bone cysts (also known as simple bone cysts or unicameral or solitary bone cysts) most commonly occur in the proximal humerus and femur, in young patients and are invariably an incidental finding. They are usually asymptomatic but if they take up a large amount of the width of the bone they can fracture and then become painful. Most cysts are left alone, but probably warrant follow up at least once to ensure that there is no change in size or symptoms. If there is any periosteal reaction further investigation is indicated to rule out malignancy or infection.

5) c.

A trigger finger is a common problem that causes pain and catching of a finger. It is usually caused by thickening of the fibrous tendon sheath, perhaps due to repetitive trauma. The condition is more common in people with diabetes and rheumatoid arthritis. As the thickened tendon sheath passes under the A1 pulley, it gets caught and can be painful. The patient often demonstrates how they can force the finger open manually using the other hand. The first line of treatment is often an injection of steroid and local anaesthetic, which may resolve things completely. Surgery involves division of the A1 pulley, which allows the tendon to glide freely without getting trapped.

EMQ 5

a. Calcaneal fracture
b. Odontoid peg fracture
c. Femoral fracture
d. Distal radial fracture
e. Osteomyelitis
f. Septic arthritis
g. Supracondylar fracture of the humerus
h. Fracture neck of femur
i. Osteosarcoma
j. Scaphoid fracture

Select the most likely diagnosis for the patients described below:

1) A 12-year-old boy who fell from a tree onto an outstretched hand and presents with a painful, flexed and swollen elbow.
2) A 32-year-old man who fell onto an outstretched hand and presents with pain in his wrist and is found to have marked tenderness in his anatomical snuffbox.
3) A 46-year-old male involved in a road traffic accident and was brought in to casualty with an open fracture, immobilised in a Thomas-Splint.
4) A 14-year-old boy who presents to his GP with a swelling in his thigh that he first noticed eight weeks ago and it now keeps him awake every night.
5) A 56-year-old lady presents with a three-month history of a painful ulcer over her heel two years after she suffered an open crush injury to this foot. Her X-ray shows periosteal reaction over the calcaneum.

Answers

1) g.

This is likely to be a supracondylar fracture of the humerus. Most of these are extension type injuries, where the distal fragment is displaced into extension leaving the sharp edge of the proximal humerus exposed and may compress or injure the brachial artery which lies just in front of it. If the fracture is non-displaced then the treatment is to flex the arm fully (checking the radial pulse). The sling provided by the triceps insertion, when the arm is fully flexed helps to stabilise the fragments. They are unstable in extension. If a supracondylar fracture is missed or the reduction is inadequate deformity can result. Angular deformities in the coronal plane do not remodel and can result in loss of the carrying angle and cubitus varus. If there is cubitus varus, internal rotation and extension of a healed supracondylar fracture this is referred to as a "gunstock deformity". Supracondylar fractures are surgical emergencies, as failure to treat vascular compromise can lead to Volkman's ischaemic contracture.

2) j.

Although a distal radial fracture is possible, the clue here is the tenderness in the anatomical snuffbox which suggests a scaphoid fracture. In undisplaced fractures, the X-ray appearance can be normal until about ten days after the injury, when the fracture line decalcifies and hence if there is a strong clinical suspicion the patient should be treated for a scaphoid fracture. An MRI scan or a bone scan can also be useful in diagnosing a scaphoid fracture. The blood supply to the scaphoid comes from distal to proximal and so in displaced fractures, the proximal pole is at risk of AVN. Undisplaced fractures can be treated conservatively in a scaphoid plaster whereas displaced fractures should be treated operatively.

3) c.

Hugh Owen Thomas developed his splint to treat femoral fractures in the late 19th century and this had a dramatic effect on reducing deaths from open femoral fractures during the First World War. It is a form of fixed traction as it relies on counter traction against the perineum by a large ring at the top of the frame. You are recommended to go to the plaster room at your hospital to see one of these splints before you sit your clinical exams as it is a prop that you could be asked about. Femoral fractures can lead to significant blood loss and there are studies that suggest stabilisation within 24 hours, reduces respiratory complications (e.g. chest infection and ARDS). One of the main factors in this is that nursing care is made easier, allowing the patients to be sat up once the fracture has been fixed. Most femoral fractures will be treated by an intramedullary nail although ORIF with plates and screws is a perfectly acceptable alternative. As the femur is such a large bone and supports so much weight they do not unite as quickly as smaller bones and it is not unusual for a femoral fracture to take between three to six months to unite in an adult.

4) i.

Any firm lump in a child that is either increasing in size, present for more than six weeks or painful at night should raise suspicion of a bony tumour. Osteosarcomas occur in males more than in females, and usually in adolescents (although there is a second peak in those over 50, due to malignant change in Paget's disease). The most common sites are around the knee or proximal humerus. Osteosarcomas usually occur in the metaphysis (the splaying end between the diaphysis and physis) and are locally invasive, spreading distally via the blood (often to the lung). Treatment usually involves chemotherapy and resection, which nowadays tends to be wide local excision using an allograft or prostheses. In certain cases, however, an amputation might be needed. About 60% survive five years.

5) e.

Following a crush injury several years ago, this lady now seems to present with an ulcer over her heel. The obvious concern is whether the infection extends into the bone, i.e. osteomyelitis. Acute osteomyelitis occurs either as a result of haematogenous spread (more common in children) or more likely in this case, following trauma/operation. In acute haematogenous osteomyelitis, the usual organisms are *Staphylococcus aureus*, but occasionally *Streptococci* or *Coliforms* are responsible. ESR is a non-specific inflammatory marker but is usually raised in osteomyelitis and the X-rays can show a periosteal reaction once the infection is established. Chronic osteomyelitis can result if a sequestrum forms. This is an area of dead bone that is walled off by new bone, often discharging through a sinus. The infection can remain for many years, giving recurrent acute flare-ups. Surgery to remove the sequestrum is indicated if healing is to ensue.

Chapter 13   Ear, Nose and Throat

Michael Oko, Ashraf Morgan and Praveen Dadireddy

Multiple Choice Questions

[Each single best answer (SBA) question comprises a stem and a number of answers. You are asked to decide which single item represents the best answer to the question.]

1. **Obstructive sleep apnoea (OSA)**

   a) Most commonly affects women over 40
   b) Is more likely in manual workers
   c) May present as snoring
   d) Surgery is a first line treatment
   e) Patients are usually asymptomatic during the daytime

[Best Answer = c]

Explanation

OSA can be defined as the combination of excessive daytime sleepiness and irregular breathing at night. Snoring, restless sleep and impaired daytime concentration are also features. The prevalence of OSA is 1%–4% but is much more common in males over 40 in sedentary occupations. The essential pathological process involved is upper airway obstruction. Lifestyle modification including weight loss, mandibular advancement devices, surgery in selected cases and CPAP are recognised treatments. The frequency of apnoea (> 10 seconds) + hypopnoea (50% reduction in tidal volume) hourly is the apnoea/hypoapnoea index and > 5 is diagnostic.

2. **Acute otitis media (OME)**

   a) Is most commonly seen in adults
   b) Usually requires surgical intervention
   c) Can cause mastoiditis and otogenic brain abscesses

d) Antibiotics should be routinely prescribed in uncomplicated OME
e) If perforation of the ear drum occurs it always needs surgical closure

[Best Answer = c]

Explanation

> Almost all children get acute OME at some stage. It usually resolves with time with or without antibiotics and antibiotics should not be routinely prescribed in uncomplicated cases. Rarely it can be complicated by spread to the cranial vault and mastoid. Most perforations of the ear drum will resolve spontaneously and do not require surgery.

3. Facial nerve

a) Gives off four branches to the face
b) Exits the temporal bone through the stylomastoid foramen
c) UMN lesions of the facial nerve affect the forehead
d) Bell's palsy is an upper motor neurone (UMN) lesion of the facial nerve
e) Full recovery is a rare occurrence in patients with Bell's palsy

[Best Answer = b]

Explanation

> It gives off five branches (temporal, zygomatic, buccal, marginal mandibular, and cervical) after passing through the stylomasoid foramen. The forehead remains mobile in UMN lesions since these muscles are supplied bilaterally. Bell's palsy, is a lower motor neurone lesion manifested as both upper and lower facial weakness on the same side of the lesion. In the majority of cases a good recovery occurs.

4. Meniere's disease — one of the following is incorrect

a) Classical symptoms are vertigo, tinnitus and deafness
b) Is almost always progressive
c) Caffeine is thought to be a trigger factor

d) Avoidance of salt may be useful

e) Gentamicin is known to be useful in the management

[Best Answer = b]

Explanation

Fluctuating pressure within the endolymphatic sac is thought to be the pathological process occurring in Ménière's and some suspect there may be an autoimmune process behind this. Avoidance of caffeine, salt and low dose diuretics are thought to be helpful. Intra-tympanic injection of gentamicin is helpful in some cases. Progression of Ménière's is unpredictable and symptoms may worsen, disappear or remain the same.

5. Larynx

a) The left recurrent laryngeal nerve loops around the subclavian artery

b) Stridor indicates noisy breathing due to obstruction at the level of the tongue base

c) Stertor means noisy respiration due to obstruction in the lower airway

d) Lymphoma is the most common malignancy of the upper airways

e) The vocal cords abduct during swallowing

[Best Answer = e]

Explanation

The right recurrent laryngeal nerve loops around the subclavian artery, the left around the arch of the aorta (ligamentum arteriosum). Stridor is a high frequency noise originating from the upper airway (trachea and larynx). Stertor is a lower frequency noise that originates from the airway above the larynx at the tongue base. Squamous cell carcinoma (SCC) is the most common malignancy of the larynx and is associated with heavy smoking. The vocal cords abduct during swallowing to prevent aspiration.

6. Foreign bodies in children

a) A foreign body in a child can be ruled out if physical examination and chest X-ray are normal

b) Mums are mostly wrong as they are often over-anxious
c) Sudden onset of stridor in a previously normal child should be considered as a foreign body unless proven otherwise
d) Organic foreign bodies can safely be left for a few months if asymptomatic
e) Acetic acid can be used to kill insects in ears

[Best Answer = c]

Explanation

> Always listen to the parent's history, as they are usually right. Endoscopy is advised in even with a negative CXR and examination if the history is strongly suggestive. Organic foreign bodies tend to swell up and should be removed as soon as possible and olive oil (not acetic acid) can be used to kill insects in the ear.

7. **Vertigo — one of the following statements is incorrect**
   a) Is usually caused by cervical spine arthritis
   b) There is often a rotatory component
   c) Benign positional vertigo is characterised by attacks of sudden onset rotational vertigo provoked by head-turning
   d) Balance during walking is principally dependent on sight
   e) URTI, vertigo and vomiting for days which settles with time suggest labyrinthitis

[Best Answer = a]

Explanation

> Vertigo is usually associated with a problem in the vestibular system, in the brain, or with the connections between these two organs. There is often a strong rotatory component to vertigo. Benign positional vertigo has the above symptoms as well as fatigability. Nystagmus can be provoked by turning the head to one side. It is thought that 70% of balance is from sight, 15% from proprioception and 15% from the vestibular system.

8. The external ear

a) When examining the ear, examine the abnormal ear first and then compare it to the normal ear
b) Endaural incision means an incision running just below the tragus
c) Accumulated wax is the most common cause for aural toileting in ENT practice
d) Otitis externa is best treated by oral antibiotics
e) Squamous carcinoma is the most common malignancy of the pinna

[Best Answer = c]

Explanation

It is traditional to examine the normal ear first and then the abnormal. Three approaches are used to operate on the external ear, endaural (anterior to the ear), Per-meatal (through the ear) and post-auricular (behind the ear). Earwax is a very common problem that can be treated with wax softeners such as olive oil, $NaHCO_3$ or syringing or microsuction. Otitis externa is best treated with aural toilet and topical antibiotics. Basal cell carcinoma is more common than squamous.

9. Acoustic neuroma — one of the following is incorrect

a) It affects the VIII cranial nerve and progressively presses on surrounding nerves and cause headaches through raised intracranial pressure
b) Known association with neurofibromatosis (NF) type II syndrome
c) Can present with unilateral sensorineural hearing loss
d) Metastasise early
e) Annual observation for growth using serial MRI is an accepted modality of management

[Best Answer = d]

Explanation

Acoustic neuromas are relatively rare, benign, slow growing lesions of the VIII CN and as they grow they cause pressure symptoms on local structures (VII) and raise intracrainial pressure (VI and headaches). In neurofibromatosis II (NF type II) you can get bilateral acoustic neuromas. In 90% there is a progressive sensorineural hearing loss associated with tinnitus in 70%. Surgery is indicated in large symptomatic lesions (> 3 cm) or rapidly growing lesions, but 60% do not show any significant annual growth. In the US sterotatic radiotherapy is popular.

10. Tinnitus

a) More commonly experienced when patient is in noisy surroundings
b) Usually experienced when patient is trying to get off to sleep
c) Is most commonly unilateral
d) Is easy to treat
e) Presents most commonly in the under 65's

[Best Answer = b]

Explanation

Tinnitus is a common condition associated with hearing loss and is most commonly perceived when the background noise is low. The origin of the word is from "ringing" but the sounds heard can vary from person to person and include buzzing, whistling as well as other sounds. But the common link is that they do not have an external source. They may be heard in one ear, both ears or centrally in the head itself. It is not a disease but a symptom associated with a wide range of underlying conditions. It can be difficult to treat and can result in sleep deprivation and depression is some patients.

11. Regarding the tympanic membrane (TM)

a) Cholesteatoma is a pre-malignant condition
b) Perforations are more common in the pars tensa segment of the TM
c) The pars flaccida is present just below the malleus
d) The light reflex is seen postero-superiorly on the TM
e) A defect in the anterior wall of the external auditory canal is indicative of a mastoid operation

[Best Answer = b]

Explanation

> Cholesteatoma is a slow growing benign epithelial cyst affecting the middle ear cleft and TM and is treated with surgery to the mastoid. The TM is divided into pars flacida above the maleus which has only two layers and pars tensa below, which has three layers. Perforations are more common in the pars tensa. The light reflex is seen antero-inferiorly on the TM and mastoid operations produce a defect in the posterior wall.

12. Glue ear — one of the following is incorrect

a) Usually occurs as a complication of acute otitis media
b) Usually seen in children between two and 11 years of age
c) Known association with allergic rhinitis
d) Can resolve spontaneously in most cases
e) Grommets are usually inserted and are left in the ear for life

[Best Answer = e]

Explanation

> All children get acute otitis media and subsequent glue ear (otitis media with effusion, OME) at some stage and this is more common around aged two years and decreases with age (1% by age 11 years). Any condition, which can cause eustachian tube dysfunction such as allergic rhinitis, can cause glue ear and in the majority of cases, it resolves spontaneously. If they is a bilateral conductive loss of > 30 db persistent for more than three months, then there is an indication to insert grommets which stay in usually between nine to 18 months before self-extruding.

13. Audiometry

a) Pure tone audiometry (PTA) is useful preliminary test in detecting acoustic neuromas
b) Clinically the 256 Hz tuning fork is used for Weber and Rinne tests
c) High frequency tuning fork causes a lot of vibrational sensation

d) Free field hearing tests are not useful clinically

e) Rinne is more sensitive than Weber's test

[Best Answer = a]

Explanation

> Asymmetrical sensorineural hearing loss can be detected with PTA which can be one of the findings in patients with acoustic neuromas. The 512 Hz tuning fork is used as it has minimal vibration and does not decay too quickly. A whispered voice at two feet is a useful and quick indicator of acceptable hearing. It is thought that Weber is a more sensitive test and will pick up losses > 5 db, while Rinne detects losses > 20 db.

14. In tonsilitis

a) Quinsy is a common complication of tonsillitis

b) Parapharyngeal abscess usually requires drainage through the oral cavity

c) Quinsy presents with trismus, otalgia and dysphagia

d) Ampicillin is the drug of choice in glandular fever

e) Tonsillectomy is indicated if there are more than two attacks in a year

[Best Answer = c]

Explanation

> Quinsy is a peritonsilar abscess that presents with trismus, otalgia and dysphagia and is drained through the oral cavity. They are quite rare nowadays because most patients get treated early. It is recommended that parapharyngeal abscesses, which are more extensive than a Quinsy, are drained through an external approach. Avoid ampicillin or drugs containing it (e.g. augumentin) if glandular fever suspected as it causes a rash. Tonsillectomy is indicated if there are more than four to six attacks in a year.

15. Otosclerosis

a) Is far more commonly seen in men
b) The inherited form usually presents in childhood
c) Usually presents with sensorineural hearing loss
d) Cannot be specifically diagnosed by an audiogram
e) Can be satisfactorily treated with a hearing aid

[Best Answer = e]

Explanation

Otosclerosis is the abnormal growth of bone in the middle ear. This causes hearing loss which may become severe. The sex incidence is about the same although females tend to present more commonly to the clinic. A family history is detectable in about half of cases and these most commonly presents between 20–30 years of age. The Carhart's notch at 2 KHz on the audiogram is classically associated with otosclerosis. A conventional hearing aid, bone anchored hearing aid or stapedectomy/stapedotomy are all recognised treatment options.

Case Studies

Case 1

An 86-year-old lady presents with a history of a longstanding lump in the front of her neck, dysphagia and stridor to the casualty department

a) What is the most likely diagnosis?
b) How should the patient be managed initially?
c) What investigations should be ordered to confirm the diagnosis?
d) What is the expected prognosis of the condition?
e) What are the main complications of the operation?

Answers

> a) A thyroid swelling — by far the most common neck lump in older females. May be malignant or benign.
> b) This is potentially life threatening. ABC approach. Secure the airway: intubation and then tracheostomy.
> c) Lateral neck and CXR, ultrasound or CT or MRI can be helpful, particularly the latter two as they can be intrathoracic extension. Histology via FNA or wedge biopsy.
> d) Depends on the histology: ranges from benign histology to lymphomas which respond well to treatment, to anaplastic carcinoma which has a 0% 12-month survival.
> e) Bleeding and haematoma, damage to recurrent laryngeal nerves, surgical emphysema, tracheomalacia, blockage or displacement of the tube.

Case 2

A frail 80-year-old patient was found after falling backwards off a train platform with blood coming out of his right ear, deafness in the right ear and vertigo

a) What is the most likely diagnosis?
b) How should the patient be managed initially?
c) What investigations should be ordered to confirm the diagnosis?

Answers

> a) Skull base fracture.
> b) ABC, manage as head injury, inform ENT department.
> c) A high resolution CT brain and temporal bone will confirm the diagnosis and detect the presence of any intracranial bleed. A pure tone audiogram with masking will detect a sensorineural or conductive hearing loss. If it is conductive it could be due to blood in the middle ear cleft or dislocation of the ossicles or a combination of both. If sensorineural the fracture line could be through the inner ear and the prognosis for recovery is poor.

Case 3

A 36-year-old lady has had a right superficial parotidectomy two weeks ago and has developed sweating and flushing over her right side of her face when she eats.

a) What is the most likely diagnosis?
b) How should the patient be managed initially?
c) What other treatment options are there?

Answers

> a) This is Frey's syndrome — a recognised complication of parotid surgery which occurs due to aberrant re-innervation between the parasympathetic and sympathetic nerve supply to the gland leading to gustatory sweating (= sweating on eating).
> b) Conservative management with reassurance (the patient should have signed a consent form pre-operatively with this, damage to the facial nerve, scar bleeding, infection and recurrence all mentioned), use make up and see if it settles with time.
> c) Tympanic neurectomy via a tympanotomy divides the parasympathetic nerve supply to the gland. Some have found that Botox injections can be helpful.

Case 4

A ten-day-old baby attends A&E with progressive stridor since birth, worse when feeding.

a) What is the most likely diagnosis?
b) How should the patient be managed initially?
c) What investigations should be ordered to confirm the diagnosis?
d) What is the expected prognosis of the condition?

Answers

a) Laryngomalacia is the most common disorder of the upper airway in children and is essentially a soft, underdeveloped cartilaginous respiratory tract, which collapses during inspiration. It can affect any and multiple parts of the respiratory tract.
b) ABC, always get consultant ENT and anaesthetic support for any airway problem, particularly with children.
c) High kV CXR outlines the respiratory tract, weight and growth charts are essential to plot progress, barium swallow rules out tracheosophageal fistulas, LA flexible nasendoscopy in theatre allows the diagnosis to be safely made and then proceed onto a GA microlarygobronchoscopy (MLB) to rule out subglottic lesions and tracheomalacia.
d) Generally good, only in extreme cases where there is a failure to thrive and persistent problems, is a tracheostomy required. With time the cartilage stiffens and the problem resolves.

Case 5

A 3-year-old non-smoking primary school teacher has a six-month history of hoarse voice.

a) What is the most likely diagnosis?
b) What investigations should be ordered to confirm the diagnosis?
c) How should the patient be managed initially?
d) What is the expected prognosis of the condition?

Answers

a) Vocal cord nodules (singer's nodules) are common with vocal abuse and classically occur at the junction of the anterior one-third and posterior two-thirds of the vocal cords at the points of maximum abrasion. Carcinoma is unlikely but should be excluded.

b) Flexible nasendocsopy in the clinic with or without local anaes-thetic provides direct visualisation of the cords and makes the diagnosis.
c) Speech and language therapy should be initially tried in combina-tion with vocal hygiene. Surgery is reserved for refractile cases.
d) Generally good.

Extended Matching Questions

EMQ 1

a. Laryngomalacia
b. Tracheo-oesophageal fistula
c. Sub-glottic stenosis
d. Foreign body
e. Laryngeal papillomatosis
f. Peanut allergy
g. Epiglottitis
h. Otitis media

For each statement below select the single most likely diagnosis:

1) Acute emergency with a drooling, unwell febrile child.
2) The most common cause of stridor in children.
3) Presents with chronic stridor and failure to thrive.
4) Presents with progressive hoarseness of voice and stridor.
5) Sudden onset of stridor in previously normal child.

Answers

1) g.
Epiglottitis (or supraglotitis). Rapid progression within hours, presents with severe odynophagia with drooling, and stridor. Presents most commonly between two to six years although can be seen in adulthood. The causative organism is usually haemophilus influenzae type B although this is changing because of the HIB vaccine, high mortality if not promptly diagnosed and treated usually managed by a team of three consultants: the otolaryngologist, anaesthetist and paediatrician. Treatment is to secure airway, take swabs for m/c/s and appropriate I.V. antibiotics.

2) a.
Approximately 60% of congenital laryngeal abnormality characterised by weak supraglottic framework which collapses on inspiration, especially during crying. It is usually self-limiting and resolves by age of three years.

3) c.

Congenital stenosis is the third most common congenital abnormality of the larynx. Acquired stenosis 90% is due to endotracheal intubation trauma. It presents with stridor during exertion or respiratory infection.

4) e.

This is the most common neoplasm of the larynx in children between two to five years and is caused by the human papilloma virus (several sub-types with different prognosis) producing warty lesions in the larynx causing hoarsness and stridor. It is treated mainly with serial laser ablation; other agents are possibly of some benefit including alpha interferon, acyclovir, and ribavirin.

5) d.

A foreign body in the airway presents with sudden onset of coughing and stridor. If neglected and lodged in a small airway the child will ultimately present with chest infection.

EMQ 2

a. Eardrum perforation
b. Parotid tumour
c. Basal cell carcinoma
d. Fractured skull
e. Chemeodectoma
f. Squamous cell carcinoma
g. Bony exostosis
h. Vestibular schwannoma (acoustic neuroma)

For each statement below select the single most likely diagnosis:

1) The most common malignant condition of external ear.
2) Commonly due to mucosal disease within middle ear cleft.
3) Usually seen in people who do a lot of swimming.
4) Malignancy that usually spreads to the deep cervical chain of lymph nodes.
5) Presents with unilateral tinnitus, vertigo or a sensorineural hearing loss.

Answers

1) c.

The most common cancer of skin in adults. Predisposing causes are UV radiation, arsenic and insecticides. BCC is a slowly growing lesion and rarely metastasis. Treated with topical agents, Mohs micrographic surgery or surgical excision with safety margin. Squamous carcinoma is the second most common.

2) a.

Tympanic membrane (= ear drum) perforation. Can be traumatic, infective or neoplastic. The most common cause is otitis media whether acute (common in children) or chronic (common in adults). TM perforation present with hearing difficulty, ear discharge and sometimes pain. Treatment of acute stage, topical antibiotics, if chronic may need surgery.

3) g.

These are firm, bony, broad-based lesions composed of lamellar bone in the bony ear canal. Formed by reactive bone formation to thermal irritation, e.g. exposure to cold water in swimming. No need for treatment usually. However if it is big it will cause wax impaction and hearing loss, which will need surgical excision of the exostosis.

4) f.

The second most common skin cancer, can be either well, moderately or poorly differentiated. Local metastasis is common to the regional lymph nodes so clinical exam and CT of regional nodes needed. Treated with surgical resection to lesion and radical neck dissection +/– radiotherapy depending on stage/spread.

5) h.

This is a slowly growing nerve sheath tumour of the superior and inferior vestibular nerves which can arise in the internal auditory canal or cerebellopontine angle. It causes symptoms by displacing, distorting and compressing adjacent structures. Treatment is observation and surgery if the tumour is progressing in size.

EMQ 3

a. Sinusitis
b. Allergic rhinitis
c. Septoplasty
d. RAST tests
e. Foreign body in nose
f. Hereditary haemorrhagic telangiectasia
g. Sphenopalatine artery ligation
h. Nasal polyps

For each statement below select the single most likely answer:

1) Autosomal dominant condition that can cause epistaxis.
2) Type I hypersensitivity reaction.
3) Treatment with antibiotics, nasal decongestants, analgesics.
4) Done for uncontrolled epistaxis.
5) Involves testing for various allergens.

Answers

1) f.
This is a capillary malformation also known as Osler-Weber-Rendu disease. It affects skin, mucous membrane, lung, liver and brain. It presents with epistaxis and GIT bleeding. Usually treated with laser ablation.

2) b.
Allergic rhinitis can be seasonal or perennial and presents with sneezing, rhinorrhea, and nasal obstruction. It may be associated with asthma, secretory otitis media, and atopic dermatitis. It can be triggered by inhaled or ingested allergens with production of IgE antibodies. Allergic rhinitis can be treated with avoidance, steroids and antihistamines.

3) a.
This is the most common disease of the paranasal sinuses. It presents with facial pain, nasal obstruction, discharge and hyposmia. Acute sinusitis responds well to antibiotics for the bacterial infection and nasal decongestant to help nasal breathing and drainage of sinuses. Chronic sinusitis may require surgery to correct anatomical variations for improving sinus drainage (functional endoscopic sinus surgery — FESS).

4) g.
Severe posterior epistaxis can be treated with arterial ligation. The sphenopalatine artery is a branch of the maxillary artery which enters the nasal cavity through the sphenopalatine foramen in the lateral wall. Ligation can be done endoscopicaly using arterial clips.

5) d.
RAST = Radioallergosorbent test, is a blood test to determine what allergens a person is allergic to. It detects the amount of IgE that react specifically to the suspected allergens.

EMQ 4

a. Benign positional vertigo
b. Tinnitus
c. Middle ear
d. Nystagmus
e. Acoustic neuroma
f. Vestibular system
g. Cholesteatoma
h. VII cranial nerve lesion

For each statement below select the single most likely answer:

1) Can be diagnosed with the Dix-Hallpike test.
2) Unilateral tinnitus may be indicative of this condition.
3) Is common in the over 65 age group and is associated with bilateral high frequency hearing loss.
4) Accounts for about 15% of the balance during walking.
5) Presents with a painless, smelly pseudomonas unilateral chronic discharge from the ear.

Answers

1) a.
Benign positional vertigo (BPPV). This is one of the most common types of peripheral vertigo, caused by debris (otoconia fragments) usually in the posterior semicircular canal. BPPV presents as sudden vertigo lasting seconds with certain head positions, no associated hearing loss. For the Dix-Hallpike test the patient is brought from the

sitting to a supine position, with the head turned 45° to one side and extended about 20° backward. The eyes are then observed for nystagmus. BPPV can be treated with repositioning manoeuvres such as Epley's manoeuvre, whereby the head is moved in such a way to cause the posterior semicircular canal to rotate around such that gravity moves the otoconia fragments out from the posterior canal and into the vestibule where they then settle and cause no symptoms.

2) e.
This is a tumour of the Schwann cells of vestibular nerve. It presents with unilateral or asymmetrical sensorineural hearing loss and/or tinnitus which can be unilateral. Investigations include audiogram, CT scan but MRI is more sensitive.

3) b.
Tinnitus. This is noises in the ears without an external source. Most commonly associated with presbycusis which is age-related sensorineural hearing loss. Tinnitus gets worse with time and usually using a hearing aid help both hearing and tinnitus.

4) f.
Balance is maintained by three sensory stimuli: vestibular, visual and proprioceptive. Stimuli are processed in the brain stem, cerebellum and cerebral cortex. Failure of any part of this system will result in imbalance and vertigo.

5) g.
This is a slow growing benign epithelial cyst affecting the middle ear cleft and tympanic membrane and usually presents with the above symptoms which can go on for years before review in the ENT department. It can be congenital or acquired and in addition to the history, examination and audiometry, high resolution CT of the temporal bones is useful in planning surgery as you can get an idea of how extensive it is before you operate. In those presenting who are not fit for surgery it can be managed in outpatients with microsuction aural toilet.

EMQ 5

a. Squamous cell carcinoma
b. Recurrent laryngeal nerve palsy
c. Acid reflux

d. Colloid goitre
e. Post-cricoid web
f. Anaplastic thyroid carcinoma
g. Retrosternal thyroid
h. Pharyngeal pouch

For each clinical scenario below select the single most likely answer:

1) An elderly patient presenting with a rapidly growing midline neck swelling, stridor and dysphagia.
2) A history of intermittent hoarse voice with globus sensation without dysphagia or weight loss.
3) Progressive dysphagia in an elderly female with a history of iron deficiency anaemia.
4) Dysphagia, otalgia, weight loss and cervical lymphadenopathy in a 65-year-old male smoker.
5) A 70-year-old man with progressive dysphagia, with food sticking at the sternal notch and regurgitation of old food and associated halitosis.

Answers

> **1 f.**
> This should always be considered as a differential diagnosis with this type of history particularly in females. Lymphoma can also present this way and the management should be to secure the airway, usually with a tracheotomy and at that time send samples for histology and get a CT from skull base to diaphragm.
>
> **2) c.**
> This is quite a common clinical cause of hoarse voice and a history of indigestion/heartburn is present in about half of cases. Nasendoscopy of the larynx reveals classic features of posterior laryngitis and usually responds to a four- to six-week course of a proton pump inhibitor (omeprazole, lansoprazole, etc.) taken about 4pm each day, with Gaviscon Advance 10–15 ml tds.
>
> **3) e.**
> This is the classic presentation seen in Brown-Kelly Patterson (Plummer-Vinson, USA) syndrome and angular stomatitis, achlorhydria in addition to the post-cricoid web. The diagnosis can be confirmed by doing the FBC reveals microcytic hypochromic anaemia in

addition to barium swallow or endoscopy. These patients are at a higher risk of carcinoma of the oesophagus, and it is more common in women than men.

4) a.

These symptoms should ring alarm bells and urgent referral to an ENT unit for full history, examination and endoscopy, biopsy, and CT skullbase to diaphragm. Single, heavy smoking and drinking males are the most common presenting group.

5) h.

Pharyngeal pouch (also known as Zenker's diverticulum in the US) is relatively rare and is a herniation at the junction of the pharynx and oesophagus in which food can collect. The aetiology is debated and is likely due to an autoimmune attack at the level of the cricopharyngeus muscle which causes spasm at this level and raised intraluminal pressure resulting in pouch formation just proximal to this. The diagnosis can be confirmed with a barium swallow or endoscopy and the management can be conservative or surgical. Endoscopic stapling is the current favoured surgical treatment although open surgery is still used for very large and revision cases. Malignancy occurs in 0.3%–1% of cases.

Chapter 14   Pre- and Post-operative Management

Ian Nesbitt and Joe Cosgrove

Multiple Choice Questions

[*Each single best answer (SBA) question comprises a stem and a number of answers. You are asked to decide which single item represents the best answer to the question.*]

1. **Criteria to diagnose the systemic inflammatory response syndrome (SIRS) include**

   a) Temperature below 36.5°C
   b) Heart rate below 90 beats per minute
   c) Respiratory rate above 17 breaths per minute
   d) White blood cell count greater than 12 or less than 4 × 10⁶
   e) Systolic blood pressure below 100 mmHg

[Best Answer = d]

Explanation

> SIRS is common after moderate and major surgery. The diagnostic characteristics are two or more of: temperature below 36°C or above 38°C; respiratory rate > 20 breaths per minute (or $PaCO_2$ below 4.3 kPa); white cell count above 12 or below $4 \times 10^6/l$; or a heart rate above 90 bpm.

2. **Acute Tubular Necrosis (ATN)**

   a) Affects the renal cortex more than medulla
   b) Impairs the function of the loop of Henlé
   c) Is part of the hepatorenal syndrome
   d) Can be caused by furosemide
   e) Decreases the clinical effect of morphine

[Best Answer = b]

Explanation

> ATN is the most common form of post-operative renal failure. It is characterised by necrosis of renal tubules (the majority of which lie in the renal medulla) including the loop of Henlé. Hepatorenal syndrome occurs in the presence of anatomically normal kidneys, and is caused by alterations in renal blood flow. High doses of furosemide can cause tubulo-interstitial nephritis. Renal failure impairs the excretion of morphine and its metabolites, thus increasing its effect. NB: it should be noted that in some patients who develop severe acute renal failure, no obvious, intrinsic damage occurs, yet the kidneys stop functioning. They effectively "shutdown" and if the body recovers, they recover. This is known as aestivation.

3. Oxygen

a) Via nasal cannulae can be delivered up to 60% inspired concentration
b) From a mask with a reservoir bag can be up to 100% inspired concentration
c) From a Venturi mask gives fixed inspired %
d) Should always be humidified
e) Is usually stored centrally in a hospital in cylinders

[Best Answer = c]

Explanation

> Nasal cannulae can deliver approximately 35% inspired oxygen concentration, while a mask and reservoir bag is more efficient and can deliver up to 80% depending on respiratory pattern. A Venturi device delivers a fixed inspired concentration of oxygen depending on which mixing device is used. Low flow oxygen rarely requires humidification, but prolonged or high flow oxygen should be humidified if possible for comfort and to prevent mucosal drying. In hospitals, oxygen is usually stored centrally in liquid oxygen tanks rather than cylinders.

4. **Regarding pulmonary thromboembolism (PTE)**

   a) PTE usually presents with haemoptysis
   b) Most patients with PTE have clinical signs of deep venous thrombosis
   c) Positive d-dimers confirm the diagnosis
   d) ECG changes of S1, Q3, T1-3 are commonly seen
   e) Computed tomography pulmonary angiography (CTPA) is the definitive investigation

[Best Answer = e]

Explanation

> PTE can present in a multitude of non-specific ways rather than just with pleuritic chest pain and haemoptysis. Only 25% of patients with PTE have clinical DVT on examination. D-Dimers are a non-specific test, so a positive result does not confirm PE, especially in the post-operative period. The classic S1Q3T3 ECG changes are, contrary to belief, in fact very rare. The definitive investigation has become CTPA, although local clinical practice may dictate that other investigations are used.

5. **Acute respiratory distress syndrome (ARDS)**

   a) Is characterised by pulmonary oedema
   b) Is always caused by sepsis
   c) Is not caused by trauma
   d) Has a mortality rate of 60%
   e) Is a contraindication to the use of steroids

[Best Answer = a]

Explanation

> ARDS is also called non-cardiogenic pulmonary oedema. Causes include burns, sepsis, trauma, pancreatitis, and pulmonary aspiration. With modern intensive care treatment (which may include steroids), the mortality rate is around 30%–40%.

6. **Which of the following drugs should not be stopped prior major surgery?**

    a) Warfarin
    b) Beta-blockers
    c) Aspirin
    d) Clopidogrel
    e) Angiotensin-2 antagonists

[Best Answer = b]

Explanation

Beta-blockers are cardioprotective and should not usually be stopped before major surgery. Warfarin has an effect that lasts several days, and is usually stopped up to a week before surgery. Depending on the type of surgery, the shorter acting heparin may be substituted until a few hours before the operation. Similarly, clopidogrel has a long duration of action and is usually stopped five to seven days pre-operatively, although in carotid endarterectomy there may be benefit in continuing the drug up to the day of surgery. Aspirin has a long duration of action, but rarely causes bleeding problems peri-operatively, so is usually stopped on the day of surgery. Angiotensin-2 antagonists can cause refractory hypotension at induction of anaesthesia, and it is usual therefore to stop them one or two days pre-operatively.

7. **The management of oliguria one day after uncomplicated left hemicolectomy starts with:**

    a) Furosemide bolus
    b) Furosemide infusion
    c) Ultrasound of renal tract
    d) Drug chart and note review
    e) Intravenous mannitol

[Best Answer = d]

Explanation

> A drug chart and clinical notes review should always be your first line of management and may reveal a particular contributing factor such as pre-existing disease, nephrotoxic drug use or surgical complication. Furosemide by infusion is more effective at producing a diuresis than the same dose given in boluses, but diuretics are infrequently required for post-operative oliguria, since the most common cause for this is hypovolaemia. Correcting the hypovolaemia, rather than forcing a diuresis (e.g. which would also be achieved with mannitol) is the correct management for most patients. Complete anuria rather than oliguria would suggest an obstructive cause requiring ultrasound examination of the renal tract (to look for a dilated system).

8. If group A negative blood is given to a group O positive recipient

a) Patients are usually initially asymptomatic
b) Patients become hypothermic rapidly
c) This is a potential cause of transfusion related death
d) Malignant hypertension occurs
e) Red cell lysis does not usually occur

[Best Answer = c]

Explanation

> Transfusing an O positive recipient with A negative blood is likely to result in a major haemolytic transfusion reaction. Symptoms of haemolytic reactions include hypotension, backache and loin pain. Haemolysis, haemoglobinuria and acute renal failure can rapidly develop. The mortality rate for this ABO incompatibility reaction is high. Urticaria and fever are common with non-haemolytic reactions.

9. Hypotension in the first post-operative day

a) Is usually due to epidural infusion of local anaesthesia
b) Is often due to dehydration
c) Is often due to inadequate analgesia

d) Is often due to the prolonged effects of anaesthetic drugs
e) Is rarely with increased capillary permeability

[Best Answer = b]

Explanation

> Hypotension is most often due to hypovolaemia, as the patient's fluid output is greater than fluid input. Pain tends to cause hypertension, and most anaesthetic drugs have a relatively short duration of action — by the time a patient returns to the ward, it is unlikely that these will cause ongoing hypotension. In addition, although an ongoing epidural infusion can cause postoperative hypotension (see Question 12), it is less common than other causes such as hypovolaemia. Hypotension can be associated with increased permeability of capillaries (especially in SIRS), and resultant leakage of fluid into the interstitial space ("third space"), causing intravascular dehydration.

10. The following are not causes of post-operative diarrhoea

a) Clostridium difficile
b) Enteral tube feeding
c) Ischaemic colitis
d) Broad-spectrum antibiotics
e) Large bowel obstruction

[Best Answer = e]

Explanation

> Aside from obstruction, all the above causes are recognised causes of diarrhoea post-operatively — C. difficile especially is increasingly associated with broad-spectrum antibiotic use. Bowel obstruction is usually associated with absolute constipation. Although diarrhoea can occur early in small bowel obstruction, it is best that you remember bowel obstruction as presenting with absolute constipation, abdominal distension and vomiting.

11. Chest drains

a) Should never have suction applied
b) Should be connected to an underwater seal, if possible
c) Should be inserted using a trocar
d) Are usually inserted in the second intercostal space in the mid-clavicular line
e) Should be angled caudally to drain a pneumothorax, and rostrally for fluid drainage

[Best Answer = b]

Explanation

An intercostal (chest) drain is usually placed in the mid-axillary line in the fifth intercostal space (emergency treatment of a tension pneumothorax includes needle thoracocentesis which is inserted into the second intercostal space in the mid-clavicular line). A chest drain is placed with blunt dissection and a finger sweep within the pleural cavity, rather than with a trocar, which in the main is a practice that has been abandoned as it is potentially very dangerous. The drain is connected to an underwater seal, and may have suction applied (typically 5–10 cm/H_2O negative pressure). Irrespective of the angle of drain insertion, both air and fluid will drain adequately.

12. Epidural analgesia

a) Causes equal sensory and motor loss when effective
b) May cause hypertension
c) May cause urinary retention
d) May cause cold feet
e) Usually delivers opiate and local anaesthetic directly into the spinal cord

[Best Answer = c]

Explanation

Drugs injected into an epidural catheter enter the epidural space, and diffuse into the subarachnoid space, spinal cord and nerve roots adjacent to the catheter. Typically, local anaesthetic and opiate combinations are used. The local anaesthetic causes a blockade of the nervous system, leading to analgesia and on occasion hypotension, vasodilation, warm feet and urinary retention. The opiate improves the quality of analgesia, but may also cause urinary retention. A sensory block is more pronounced than a motor block, since the anaesthetic diffuses into the smaller, unmyelinated (and less myelinated) pain fibres more readily than the large, myelinated motor fibres. Patients often find motor block to be disquieting and unpleasant. (Note: a dense motor block may indicate cord injury from an epidural haematoma — an emergency requiring rapid identification, ideally via magnetic resonance imaging (MRI)).

13. Type 2 diabetic patients

a) Should have peri-operative blood glucose controlled between 8–12 mmol/l
b) Have high incidence of post-operative complications even following minor procedures
c) Should be placed near the start of an operating list
d) Are usually not suitable for day case surgery
e) Should omit oral hypoglycaemic agents for two days pre-operatively

[Best Answer = c]

Explanation

Diabetics should ideally have glucose level controlled between 5–9 mmol/l — peri-operatively. With good control, complication rates should be similar to other patients for most types of surgery. Logistically, it is best to place diabetic patients near the start of a list to avoid prolonged fasting and possible hypoglycaemia pre-operatively. Many procedures can be carried out on a day-case basis, and frequently, patients can take their normal medication until the morning of surgery, when it should be omitted as the patient is starved.

14. Pulse Oximetry

a) Is not related to peripheral perfusion
b) Is a good indicator of ventilatory ability
c) Measures the absolute amount of saturated haemoglobin
d) May be inaccurate in heavy smokers
e) Is inaccurate in pigmented skin

[Best Answer = d]

Explanation

> Pulse oximetry measures the ratio of desaturated to saturated haemo-globin, and usually displays this as a percentage saturation spec-trophotometric trace (SpO_2), along with heart rate. Poor peripheral perfusion is a common cause of low SpO_2. Pulse oximetry measures oxygenation, not ventilation, so is not a good single monitor for res-piratory function. In fact, under certain circumstances (such as brain-stem death testing) it is possible for a patient to remain apnoeic (i.e. no ventilation) for a significant time before oxygenation is affected. Carboxyhaemoglobin (as in heavy smokers or burn victims) causes inaccuracies, but pigmented skin usually does not.

15. The following investigations are appropriately matched with the clinical presentation

a) Laparotomy for persistent upper gastrointestinal bleeding 24 hours after sclerotherapy of oesophageal varices
b) Selective angiography for torrential lower gastrointestinal bleeding in a patient with angiodysplasia
c) Selective angiography for recurrent minor lower gastrointestinal bleeding in patient with angiodysplasia
d) Colonoscopy for melaena 24 hours after sclerotherapy for bleeding oesophageal varices.
e) Abdominal ultrasound for profuse offensive diarrhoea with painful abdom-inal distension after prolonged antibiotic treatment

[Best Answer = b]

Explanation

Oesophageal varices often re-bleed despite initial interventions such as sclerotherapy or banding. Gastroscopy is appropriate to confirm and treat any ongoing bleeding point, not a laparotomy. Altered blood from a proximal bleeding site can be passed per rectum for several days afterwards, and does not usually require investigation unless there is evidence of ongoing bleeding. Angiography is a useful investigation and intervention in the setting of GI bleeding, but the volume of bleeding needs to be significant (often values of 200 ml/min are quoted), especially if colonoscopy is not possible due to the volume of blood loss. Abdominal pain and diarrhoea after antibiotic treatment should raise the possibility of toxic megacolon and hence require an abdominal X-ray (note: it could also indicate *Clostridium difficile* infection).

Case Studies

Case 1

A 60-year-old man with liver disease is admitted for routine hip replacement, and develops an acute confusional state three days post-operatively, with hypertension, tachycardia, hyperthermia, and profound sweating. His pre-operative medication includes chlordiazepoxide, phenytoin and dothiepin.

a) What is the most likely diagnosis from the information given?
b) What other important diagnoses should be considered?
c) What is the appropriate management?
d) What is the non-pharmacological management?
e) What drugs may be helpful?
f) How can you assess the degree of confusion?

Answers

a) Delirium Tremens. This is an acute organic disorder caused by cessation of chronic alcohol consumption. Clinical features include confusion, delirium, delusions and hallucinations, tremor, agitation, insomnia and signs of autonomic hyperactivity (e.g. elevated blood pressure and heart rate, dilated pupils, and sweating).

b) Other organic causes, especially infection (e.g. chest, urinary tract); metabolic abnormalities (e.g. hypoglycaemia, hyponatraemia); other drug withdrawal; and myocardial infarction.

c) As with all cases, you need to elicit as much of the relevant history from the patient as possible; carry out a full physical examination; and then investigate as directed by the findings in your history and examination. In this case, the relevant tests would include an infection screen. The following would be a reasonable batch of tests: a BM Stix, urine culture and blood tests (e.g. full blood count, urea electrolytes and blood glucose). If you had a strong suspicion of septicaemia, you would also send blood cultures.

d) Treat the cause plus environmental control; use of experienced nursing staff to prevent further agitation or harm.

e) Appropriate sedation/antipsychotics (frequently chlordiazepoxide for alcohol withdrawal, plus haloperidol). Consider Thiamine and B vitamins.

Case 2

A 60-year-old man is admitted for bowel surgery. Routine enquiry reveals that he has had several pre-syncopal episodes in the previous month. He had a permanent pacemaker inserted for similar episodes a number of years previously. His ECG is shown below.

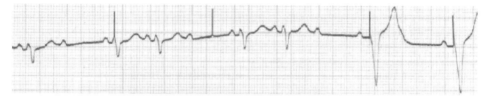

a) What does this show?
b) What may cause this?
c) What other symptoms may be reported?
e) What are four relevant questions to ask about the pacemaker?
e) What three other tests are required?
f) Who should be informed about the pacemaker?
g) What problems can arise in theatre if this had not been identified?
h) Does this patient require prophylactic antibiotics against endocarditis?

Answers

a) A malfunctioning ventricular pacemaker with an underlying natural rhythm of second degree heart block (Mobitz). P wave 1 (P1) is normally conducted, with a natural ventricular beat produced. P2 and P8 are non-conducted beats. P3 is normal, as is its associated ventricular response, although the pacemaker generates an inappropriate pacing spike (S1). P4, 6 and 7 are normal, P5 is non-conducted, and S2 fails to capture the ventricle. P9 and P10 are appropriately activating pacing spikes causing paced ventricular beats.

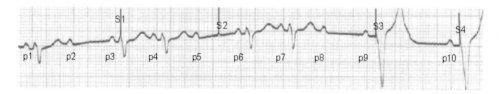

b) Usually due to lead fracture or displacement; battery failure; or metabolic abnormalities.

c) Brady or tachycardia; missed beats/palpitations; or hiccups. Occasionally, symptoms relating to permanent pacemaker (PPM) infection may be reported, such as inflammation over the pacing box, purulent discharge or systemic symptoms, e.g. fever.

d) Why was it inserted? When was it inserted? What sort of pacemaker is it? Is it working properly?

e) Chest X-ray (to look for lead fracture); pacemaker function test; urea and electrolytes.

f) The anaesthetist should be told about the pacemaker problem. The pacemaker clinic should also be informed so they can organise a PPM test.

g) Surgical diathermy may reset or damage a PPM. Temporary pacing may be required. Other implantable devices such as defibrillators may also be affected by diathermy.

h) No. The British National Formulary (BNF) contains current recommendations for endocarditis prophylaxis.

Case 3

A 67-year-old man suffers the sudden onset of tachycardia, hypotension and respiratory distress with central chest pain, four days following a Whipple's procedure (pancreaticoduodenal resection) for carcinoma of the head of pancreas. His medical history includes a deep venous thrombosis and stable angina

a) What are four important diagnoses to consider?

b) His ECG is shown below. List two abnormalities and the most likely diagnosis.

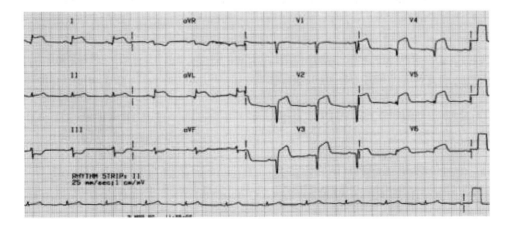

c) What other investigations may help confirm the diagnosis?
d) What are the immediate possible treatments for this condition?
e) What are other possible early treatments and are any of these contraindicated for this man?
f) What follow up investigations should this man have after this acute phase?
g) Which coronary artery is most likely to be involved?

Answers

a) Acute coronary syndrome (ACS) or myocardial infarction; pulmonary thromboembolism (PTE); pneumonia; sepsis from subphrenic collection is also possible, but less likely than the first three diagnoses.

b) Widespread anterolateral ST elevation and inferior ST depression suggests acute anterior myocardial infarction and inferior ischaemia (although the latter may represent reciprocal changes only).

c) Cardiac enzymes (troponin I, troponin T, or CK-MB); serial ECG; and arterial blood gases. A CT pulmonary angiogram may be required to exclude PTE.

d) Oxygen, aspirin, β blockers, nitrates, opiate analgesia, antiemetics. Anti-coagulation carries risks in the immediate post-operative period, and should be discussed with senior colleagues.

e) Percutaneous coronary intervention (PCI) with stent or antiplatelet agents, statins, ACE inhibitors if impaired cardiac function. Intravenous thrombolysis is probably contraindicated in view of recent surgery, and the significant contrast load involved in PCI may be a concern if renal function is poor. ACE inhibitors may be contraindicated if renal function is poor.

f) Echocardiography. Consider exercise stress testing and angiography.

g) Without angiography, it is difficult to say, but in most people, the left anterior descending artery (LAD) supplies the anterolateral myocardium, apex, and interventricular septum. The posterior descending artery PDA (usually a branch of the right coronary artery, but often a branch of the left circumflex artery) supplies the inferior wall, ventricular septum, and the posteromedial papillary muscle. In this patient, the anterolateral infarction is most likely caused by occlusion of the LAD.

Case 4

A 45-year-old man with learning difficulties is found collapsed on the ward one evening. His notes are missing, but the nursing staff say that he had an uneventful varicose vein procedure two days previously, and was due to go home the next day. Examination reveals he is unconscious (GCS 4/15), with no focal neurological abnormalities or obvious injuries. His HR is 70 bpm and BP 140/70. SpO₂ is 98%, Respiratory rate 20 bpm, Temperature 36.8°C.

a) What are the immediate management priorities?
b) What are the three most likely diagnoses?
c) What immediate tests are required?
d) What else should you do?
e) Does he require endotracheal intubation?
f) What other imaging may be important?
g) Who should transfer this patient to the radiology suite (if required)?

Answers

a) ABC's — Airway management (including provision of oxygen), breathing and circulation assessment and management. It is also important to get help, rather than attempting to manage complex and emergency cases alone.

b) Hypoglycaemia, epilepsy, simple faint.

c) Check glucose using a BM stix; send blood for urea and electrolytes, full blood count and blood glucose.

d) Get his notes and drug kardex, and speak with his supervising team to gain additional information.

e) It depends on the cause: assuming he is spontaneously breathing and the cause is a rapidly correctable condition such as hypoglycaemia, a single epileptic fit, or a simple faint, then placing him in the recovery position may be sufficient. Intubation may be required if he does not recover quickly.

f) CT Head is perhaps the most useful additional imaging in this case. Radiography of his cervical spine and chest is unlikely to be beneficial given the history and physical findings.

g) In the UK, anaesthetists should be involved in transport to the radiology department for CT Head. Most recommendations suggest that patients with a Glasgow Coma Score of 8 or less require intubation and mechanical ventilation for airway protection during transfer for imaging studies or ongoing care. The situation may vary in other healthcare systems.

Case 5

A 60-year-old man with chronic obstructive lung disease and moderate renal failure (due to renovascular disease) is admitted for renal angiography. He suffers a femoral artery false aneurysm requiring formal surgical repair under general anaesthesia. Two days later, he is tachypnoeic, hypoxaemic and distressed. His arterial blood gases (ABG) and chest X-ray (CXR) are shown below.

FiO_2: 0.5; pH 7.33; $PaCO_2$ 4.1 kPa; PaO_2 8.7 kPa; HCO_3 22 mmol/l; base excess — 2.3 mmol/l.

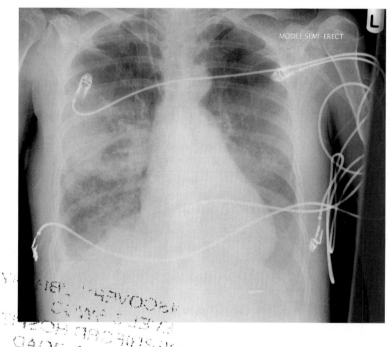

a) What abnormalities do the ABG show?
b) List three abnormalities on the CXR.
c) What is the most likely diagnosis?
d) List two possible underlying causes for this.
e) What is the immediate management?
f) What other investigations will be immediately helpful?
g) What other management options should be considered?

Answers

a) Type 1 respiratory failure (marked hypoxaemia with normal PaCO$_2$) and a mild metabolic acidosis.

b) Blunting of costophrenic angles, enlarged pulmonary vasculature, increased airspace shadowing (especially in right mid zone), and pulmonary oedema can be seen. A nasogastric tube, central line and ECG wires are also visible. One cannot comment on heart size (since this is a semi-erect AP film).

c) Acute pulmonary oedema — less likely in this context are pneumonia or atelectasis.

d) Acute myocardial infarction or acute lung injury/ARDS (less likely).

e) Airway (with Oxygen), Breathing, Circulation; get help.

f) ECG and cardiac enzymes.

g) Nitrates, blood pressure control, diuretics, aspirin and possibly ACE inhibitors. Continuous positive airway pressure (CPAP) — usually requires admission to the critical care unit. Further investigations of cardiac function should also be considered.

Extended Matching Questions

EMQ 1

a. Acute myocardial infarction
b. Pulmonary thromboembolism (PTE)
c. Tension pneumothorax
d. Bronchopneumonia
e. Costochondritis
f. Pericarditis
g. Haemothorax
h. Oesophageal rupture
i. Mediastinitis
j. Thoracic aortic dissection

Match the most probable diagnosis with the information below:

1) Seventy-year-old man with chest pain two days after emergency infrarenal aortic aneurysm repair.
2) Thirty-year-old man with postural related chest pain two days after blunt trauma to the chest. On examination a pericardial friction rub is heard.
3) Forty-five-year-old man dyspnoeic one hour after central venous catheter insertion.
4) Forty-five-year-old man with blood-stained sputum and collapse ten days after pelvic surgery.
5) Forty-five-year-old male smoker with productive cough five days after abdominal surgery.

Answers

Several of the diagnoses might be correct, but the key is to decide which is the most likely (i.e the best answer).

1) a.
Aortic aneurysm is often associated with coronary artery disease, and emergency repair is a major physiological insult that has a significant likelihood of causing myocardial ischaemia and infarction. In fact myocardial infarction is the most common cause of death after technically successful aneurysm repair.

2) f.
Pericarditis has a variety of causes, including chest trauma. Classically, this pain is worse when leaning forwards.

3) c.
Central line insertion carries a risk of pneumothorax. The onset of symptoms may be delayed by several hours. This is a more common complication than haemothorax.

4) b.
Blood-stained sputum is one of the symptoms of PTE. Pelvic surgery is a significant risk factor for PTE. Classically, PTE occurs ten days post-operatively, although there is wide variation in real life. Collapse and cardiogenic shock due to obstruction of blood flow through the pulmonary tree can be fatal.

5) d.
A productive cough after abdominal surgery is frequently due to a chest infection following poor mobilisation and inadequate clearance of secretions.

EMQ 2

a. D-Dimers
b. CT pulmonary angiography
c. Radiocontrast swallow
d. Ultrasound chest
e. Electrocardiography
f. Chest X-ray
g. Bronchoscopy
h. Duplex ultrasound of leg veins
i. Gallium labelled white cell scan
j. Ventilation perfusion scan

Choose the best initial diagnostic test for the cases below:

1) Thirty-year-old man with Boerhave's syndrome.
2) Seventy-year-old man with chest pain one day after elective infrarenal aortic aneurysm repair.
3) Forty-five-year-old patient with rheumatoid arthritis and a suddenly tender, swollen calf ten days after bowel surgery.

4) Forty-five-year-old with non-productive cough and fever seven days after major surgery.

5) Forty-five-year-old with severe dyspnoea, pleuritic chest pain, blood tinged sputum and fever seven days after major surgery.

Answers

1) c.
Boerhave's syndrome is a ruptured oesophagus (typically after prolonged vomiting). It carries a high mortality rate especially if diagnosis is delayed. A water soluble (e.g. gastrograffin) swallow is the investigation of choice.

2) e.
Chest pain after aortic surgery requires exclusion of myocardial ischaemia, although as time passes, other diagnoses may become more likely.

3) h.
Patients with rheumatoid arthritis are at risk of a deep vein thrombosis and hence a duplex ultrasound is indicated to rule out proximal extension of a thrombosis (note: duplex is not good at assessing the veins below the knee but is accurate for above knee DVTs). Also it can diagnose a ruptured Baker's cyst, which is more common in rheumatoid patients).

4) f.
A non-productive cough with fever one week after surgery is a non-specific presentation, and a chest X-ray is a reasonable initial investigation.

5) b.
Blood-stained sputum with severe dyspnoea a week after surgery is suggestive of pulmonary embolism and the investigation of choice in this situation would be CT pulmonary angiography.

EMQ 3

a. Diabetic ketoacidosis (DKA)
b. Insulinoma
c. Hyper-osmolar non-ketotic coma (HONK)
d. Cushing's disease
e. Addisonian crisis
f. Conn's syndrome
g. Phaeochromocytoma
h. Urinary tract infection (UTI)
i. Cushing's syndrome
j. Subphrenic abscess

What is the most appropriate diagnosis for the presenting scenarios?

1) Cardiovascular collapse in a patient with chronic severe rheumatoid disease three days after hip replacement surgery.
2) Patient with intractable hypertension and hypokalaemia admitted for elective adrenal surgery.
3) Patient with neurofibromatosis and paroxysmal hypertension admitted for elective adrenal surgery.
4) Patient with history of polyuria and recurrent skin abscesses, now admitted confused, with an acute abdomen.
5) Patient with hypertension, obesity, hyperglycaemia and visual field defect presenting for neurosurgery.

Answers

> **1) e.**
> Rheumatoid arthritis is often treated with steroids, and long term use can cause adrenal suppression. The stress of surgery can trigger an Addisonian crisis. This classically presents with hypotension, confusion, weakness and nausea and vomiting with abdominal or back pain. Unrecognised and untreated, it carries a high mortality rate.
>
> **2) f.**
> Conn's syndrome is primary hyperaldosteronism, due to a tumour of the adrenal cortex. Intractable hypertension, hypernatraemia and hypokalaemia are part of the clinical picture of this uncommon disease. Whilst Cushing's disease (pituitary tumour) and Cushing's

syndrome (steroid excess) present with similar biochemistry (and impaired glucose tolerance), they are less likely to have an intra-abdominal cause.

3) g.

Neurofibromatosis (also known as Von Recklinghausen's disease) is associated with phaeochromocytoma, which, along with Conn's syndrome, is one of the uncommon causes of hypertension amenable to surgical excision.

4) a.

Polyuria and recurrent infections may be due to hyperglycaemia in poorly controlled diabetes. This is also a recognised non-surgical cause of an acute abdomen.

5) d.

A pituitary tumour may cause visual field defects due to its proximity to the optic chiasm. Classically, this is a bitemporal hemianopia. Cushing's disease is due to an excess of adrenocorticotrophin hormone causing over-activity of the adrenal cortex.

Frequently, the clinical picture of endocrine disorders is not classical, and some overlap in presentation can occur. Specific and sometimes recurrent investigation may be required to make the correct diagnosis.

EMQ 4

a. Cryoprecipitate
b. Fresh frozen plasma (FFP)
c. Packed red cells
d. Whole blood
e. O-negative blood
f. Type-specific blood
g. No intervention
h. Vitamin K
i. Platelets
j. Corticosteroids

Match the most appropriate treatment with the disease state below:

	Disease State	Hb (g/dl)	Plt (× 10¹²/l)	PT (sec)	APTT (sec)	Fibrinogen (g/dl)
	(Normal Values)	(12.2–17.5)	(150–400)	(16–18)	(25–35)	(2–4)
1)	Patient with liver disease requiring urgent central line insertion	9.8	101	22	32	3.3
2)	Cardiovascular stable patient one hour following TURP	6.7	388	15	35	2.6
3)	Major obstetric haemorrhage with cardiovascular instability	3.2	246	16	40	4.7
4)	Severe sepsis	9.5	55	17	36	0.3
5)	Warfarinised for aortic valve replacement	12.9	310	36	34	1.8

Answers

> *Normal (reference) values for haematological tests vary with age, sex and the population under consideration. It is useful to learn reference values for common tests. Several of the options a–j may be reasonable for cases 1–5, but are frequently situation dependent. The most accepted in current UK practice are mentioned, with explanations where appropriate for other options.*

1) b.

Liver disease alters vitamin K-dependent clotting enzymes. Often, liver disease is associated with a high PT. Both vitamin K and FFP would be reasonable, but often FFP is used for invasive procedures such as liver biopsy or central line insertion, since its onset of action is immediate. If FFP was unavailable (or contraindicated), or if this patient had a less severe coagulopathy, or was awaiting a less urgent procedure, vitamin K would be a suitable option (although it may take several days to see the full effects).

2) c.

TURP is associated with non-compressible haemorrhage (from the prostatic venous plexus). Transfusion of red blood cells is indicated for significant bleeding. In UK practice, this most commonly involves packed red cells for patients who are physiologically stable. If a coagulopathy develops, other blood products may be required. If the patient was physiologically unstable, type-specific or O-positive may become reasonable choices.

3) e.

Major obstetric haemorrhage with cardiovascular instability is life-threatening. In UK practice, the quickest way to give blood is to use O-negative blood (the universal donor), rather than waiting for a formal cross-match. Type-specific blood may be an option if the patient is more stable. Other healthcare systems may have alternatives (such as haemoglobin carrying blood substitute solutions).

4) a.

In severe sepsis, disseminated intravascular coagulopathy can develop. The management of this complex disease frequently requires multiple different blood products. In this case, the anaemia, thrombocytopaenia and prolonged PT/APTT are not severe enough to require immediate intervention. Although corticosteroids are used in sepsis to improve cardiovascular function, and have a beneficial effect on platelet function when used chronically, the principal concern in this scenario is the low fibrinogen level, which should be treated with cryoprecipitate.

5) g.

Warfarin predominantly affects the prothrombin time (PT). A PT double or triple normal (INR of 2–3) is a common therapeutic goal for treatment and hence this is a deliberate set of appropriate blood values requiring no intervention.

EMQ 5

a. Wound dehiscence
b. Ischaemic colitis
c. Intestinal infarction
d. Superficial wound infection

e. Resolving haematoma
f. Gastroparesis
g. Acute pancreatitis
h. Bleeding peptic ulcer
i. Empyema of gall bladder
j. Ascending cholangitis

Match the most likely post-operative complication with the procedure:

1) Fresh rectal bleeding with diarrhoea 36 hours after repair of ruptured aortic aneurysm.
2) Jaundice four days after ruptured aortic aneurysm repair, with normal gamma glutamyl transferase (γGT).
3) Atrial fibrillation and severe central abdominal pain with acidosis 24 hours after cardiac surgery.
4) Inflamed mid-line laparotomy with gaping wound edges and sero-sanguinous fluid leakage.
5) Rigours associated with jaundice 12 hours after ERCP and sphincterotomy for gallstones.

Answers

1) b.
Acute bowel ischaemia often presents with bloody diarrhoea. Although this is an uncommon complication of aneurysm repair, it is important to identify early (before perforation and peritonitis set in). The ischaemia tends to affect the mucosa rather than the full thickness of the bowel wall.

2) e.
Jaundice will result if the capacity of the liver to process bilirubin is overcome (e.g. large haematoma breakdown). GGT is a sensitive marker, especially of cholestatic liver disease, and jaundice in the presence of a normal level of GGT is unlikely to be due to an obstructive cause.

3) c.
Atrial fibrillation is a common arrhythmia after cardiac surgery, and is a risk factor for superior mesenteric artery embolism (the most common cause of acute small bowel infarction). Often, bowel ischaemia is a difficult diagnosis to make, and has a high mortality rate.

4) a.

A superficial wound infection can progress to wound dehiscence, which is the separation of a surgical wound. Typically, pink sero-sanguinous fluid leakage is more suggestive of a dehiscence rather than a simple wound infection. Dehiscence may be relatively superficial or, more impressively, can involve the whole abdomen bursting open.

5) j.

One of the complications of ERCP/sphincterotomy is ascending cholangitis — infection within an obstructed biliary tree.